RECLAIMING BREASTFEEDING FOR THE UNITED STATES

Protection, Promotion, and Support

Karin Cadwell, Ph.D., R.N., I.B.C.L.C.

WITH

Cindy Turner-Maffei, M.A., I.B.C.L.C.

Anna Blair, Ph.D.

Lois Arnold, M.P.H., I.B.C.L.C.

Zoë Maja McInerney, M.A., C.L.C.

Charles Cadwell, Ph.D.

Kajsa Brimdyr, Ph.D.

JONES AND BARTLETT PUBLISHERS

Sudbury, Massachusetts

BOSTON   TORONTO   LONDON   SINGAPORE

World Headquarters
Jones and Bartlett Publishers
40 Tall Pine Drive, Sudbury, MA 01776
978-443-5000
info@jbpub.com
www.jbpub.com

Jones and Bartlett Publishers Canada
2406 Nikanna Road
Mississauga, ON L5C 2W6, CANADA

Jones and Bartlett Publishers International
Barb House, Barb Mews
London W6 7PA, UK

Library of Congress Cataloging-in-Publication Data

Reclaiming breastfeeding for the United States : protection, promotion and support / Karin Cadwell, editor; with Cindy Turner-Maffei . . . [et al.].
        p. cm.
    Includes bibliographical references and index.
    ISBN 0-7637-2096-8
    1. Breast feeding promotion—United States. 2. Breast feeding—United States. 3. Breast feeding—Social aspects-United States. 4. Infants—United States-Nutrition. I. Cadwell, Karin. II. Turner-Maffei, Cindy.

RJ216 .R34 2002
649'.33'0973-dc21

                                                                2001050738

Acquisitions Editor: Penny M. Glynn
Associate Editor: Thomas Prindle
Production Manager: Amy Rose
Manufacturing Buyer: Amy Duddridge
Typesetting: Carlisle Publishers Services
Cover Design: Philip Regan
Printing and Binding: Malloy Lithographing

Printed in the United States of America

06 05 04 03 02 10 9 8 7 6 5 4 3 2 1

CONTENTS

FOREWORD

Will It Ever Be American to Breastfeed?

Human lactation has sustained humankind since Adam and Eve, but breastfeeding has been a topic of interest only to mothers and their babies and their lay support friends and family. In the early 20th century as technology began to evolve, it became practical and safe to bottle feed infants with the discovery of the significance of sterilization to infant morbidity and mortality, and the ability to sterilize formulas at home. Bottles and nipples were available in the marketplace and physicians concocted their own brand of special feeding for newborns. Gradually, this personalized feeding was replaced by the standardization of evaporated milk formulas and the availability of dextro maltose and karo syrup to provide additional carbohydrates. In the 1930s and 1940s, the science of infant formula production evolved and infant formulas became available in the grocery store rather than at the pharmacy. Gradually, breastfeeding disappeared and medical practitioners encouraged the use of these scientific formulas. Furthermore, mothers became interested in raising their infants by the book and scientifically, which implied the use of artificial feeding mechanisms.

In 1945, Edith B. Jackson, a pediatrician and self-designed psychiatrist on the faculty at Yale University School of Medicine, obtained a five-year grant in cooperation with the Department of Obstetrics at Yale to initiate a new approach to childbirth and child-rearing. This was called the rooming-in project, and a key piece included the maintaining of the mother and baby side-by-side in a special unit where a nursing staff took care of mother and baby couples. An important corollary of this program was prepared childbirth, and Dr. Jackson initiated the American version of childbirth without fear, originally developed by Grantley Dick Reid in England. This involved prenatal classes and preparation for childbirth. The other major goal in the rooming-in project was to encourage women to breastfeed. Dr. Jackson and her colleagues published the first medical document on the management of breastfeeding in 1952 based on the follow-up of hundreds of breastfeeding mothers and babies. A report of this work appeared in the *Journal of the American Medical Association* and was widely copied, but rarely credited, as interest in breastfeeding slowly developed among professional and lay groups. Dr. Jackson's program continued through the 1950s and became a permanent hallmark of obstetrical and neonatal care at Yale University. Every resident who completed the training in obstetrics and pediatrics at Yale during those years had to spend time in the rooming-in unit and was required to make home visits in follow-up of breastfeeding management of their patients. Many very insightful articles emanated from this program as breastfeeding was studied by a generation of postgraduate fellows in Dr. Jackson's program.

In the late 1950s, a small band of seven young mothers all nursing their infants met at a picnic in Illinois and planted the seed from which the mighty oak, La Leche League International, has grown as a world-wide mother-to-mother program to support breastfeeding. Medical interest in breastfeeding did not grow so rapidly and many of Dr. Jackson's students spread out across the country and developed their own programs wherever they chose to practice. The first great breakthrough in attracting national attention to the issues of breastfeeding came in 1984 when Dr. C. Everett Koop, then Surgeon General of the United States, requested that the breastfeeding researchers at the University of Rochester develop a Surgeon General's Workshop to investigate the major issues of encouraging and increasing breastfeeding in the United States.

Dr. Koop stated that "We must identify and reduce barriers which keep women from beginning or continuing to breastfeed their infants." The deliberations and recommendations were categorized into common themes and were reported under the following six headings: (1) World of Work; (2) Public Education; (3) Professional Education; (4) Health-Care System; (5) Support Services; and (6) Research.

Commitment to the recommendations were backed by Dr. Koop with personal effort and federal funds. The American Academy of Pediatrics and the American College of Obstetrics & Gynecology responded to the challenge by strengthening their mandate to their members. A work group on breastfeeding was established by the A.A.P. and the landmark statement about breastfeeding was published in 1997, stating that an infant should be exclusively breastfeeding for six months, continue breastfeeding while adding solid foods until a year of age, and then as long thereafter as mother and infant wish.

In the decade that followed the workshop, a new specialty developed—the International Board Certified Lactation Consultant (I.B.C.L.C.), who was certified by the International Board of Lactation Consultant Examiners. The consultant was enabled to establish a practice. This encouraged non-medical practitioners to establish practices. Other terms for specialist were created and other training programs offered other recognition based on participation in special programs. The I.B.C.L.C. examination is offered annually in at least 20 countries and more than eight languages.

The Academy of Breastfeeding Medicine (A.B.M.) was founded in 1993 as an international organization for physicians who needed a forum to encourage, promote, and support breastfeeding.

A major step toward national commitment for breastfeeding occurred with the development of the United States Breastfeeding Committee, a national not-for-profit organization of organizations. That is, membership is by representation of organizations significantly committed to breastfeeding such as the American Academy of Pediatrics, the American College of Obstetrics & Gynecology, the American Academy of Family Practice, and 30 other professional organizations. The purpose of this committee is to further the breastfeeding agenda and assist and support the Surgeon General, the Bureau of Maternal and Child Health, and Women, Infants, & Children Nutrition Program (W.I.C.) to increase the incidence and duration of breastfeeding, especially among national and ethnic groups who currently do not breastfeed in any great numbers.

As more and more interest has been generated around breastfeeding, more and more information has appeared in medical, nursing, and lay literature on the topic. A major dilemma for the consumer is sorting out the deluge of scientific work from the anecdotal information that emanates from folklore or experimental authority. This volume lays a firm foundation for understanding the issues in the United States today. It describes the Baby-Friendly Hospital Initiative impact on hospital practice behavior and reviews the impact of breastfeeding in the health care system. Discussion of evidence-based breastfeeding practice brings to the reader's attention the need to evaluate the literature carefully and to select only that material done by reputable investigators in a scientifically controlled, statistically valid manner. Additional time is given to recommendations for overcoming the disparities in breastfeeding between various ethnic, cultural, and social groups. Very importantly, the issue of human milk being provided for very sick and premature infants in neonatal intensive care units who cannot initially feed directly at the breast is detailed. The role of banked donor milk is also addressed. This is a significant issue for many babies in the hospital and outside and has become a technical challenge in this era of HIV and hepatitis infections.

As noted in the introduction, this book is not a general reference about breastfeeding or instructions for nursing a child. It is, on the other hand, about where breastfeeding is going in the United States, how much has been accomplished, and all the work that is yet to be done. The work that is yet to be done includes changing hospital policy as advocated by the Baby-Friendly Hospital Initiative, educating health care professionals more fully in the fields of breastfeeding and human lactation, and developing a reliable, readily available, economic source for human milk available for those infants with special needs whose mothers cannot provide a sufficient supply. A national commitment of funds and a federal policy of support are the mandatory underpinnings of the process of "Reclaiming Breastfeeding for the United States."

Ruth A. Lawrence, M.D.
Professor of Pediatrics, Obstetrics & Gynecology
University of Rochester School of Medicine

ACKNOWLEDGMENTS

The completion of a project as complex as this book is reason for celebration. The work of writing and the ongoing work of reclaiming breastfeeding builds on the wisdom and creativity of colleagues and researchers too numerous to list here, although our gratitude is unbounded. Thank you.

The Authors

INTRODUCTION

This book is not a general reference about breastfeeding, nor does it attempt to help a woman breastfeed her child. It will not serve as a reference for breastfeeding problems. Rather, this book is about the progress we have made in the United States health care system toward reclaiming breastfeeding as the normal way to feed babies and young children. It is also about the work we have yet to do. As the United States continues to integrate and reengineer health care services, the significance of breastfeeding initiation, exclusivity, and duration to the community increases. The exact value of breastfeeding in terms of financial benefit to the system is unknown, but it is acknowledged to be important both in short-term savings (for example, costs of office visits and prescriptions in the first year of life) and long-term costs for identified chronic diseases. As the United States works to change the health care paradigm from one in which ill health results in increased profit to one in which health promotion and healthy behaviors seek to reduce costs, breastfeeding becomes one of the key strategies for improved health.

Like so many other projects before it, this project turned out to be considerably more complicated and more rewarding than we ever imagined. Writing this book was a process of discovery. We started with asking and answering the questions: "How did we get to this point in the political and economic history of breastfeeding?" and "What can we learn for the future?" We saw clearly what has been accomplished in the United States compared to our goals, which propelled additional thought about complexities in the U.S. health care system. We examined the issue of reclaiming breastfeeding in the United States from different aspects. We looked at political forces, studies published in professional literature, our practices, and our own experience. We asked the questions: "What has already worked in the U.S. health care system to reclaim breastfeeding?" and "What more can be done to implement comprehensive, current, and culturally appropriate lactation care and services for all women and their nursing infants and growing children?"

Our Process

The analysis of reclaiming breastfeeding in the United States involved a multimethod research approach called "crystallization." According to Morse:

> Because different "lenses" or perspectives result from the use of different methods, often more than one method may be used within a project so the researcher can gain a more holistic view . . . provided the analysis is kept separate and not muddled.[1]

Multimethod research is often called "triangulation," but: "[i]n post-modern mixed-genre texts we do not 'triangulate'; we crystallize. We recognize that there are far more than 'three sides' from which to approach the world."[2] The methods we used to crystallize our ideas included writing as inquiry, integrative research review, combinational analysis, and qualitative analysis of interviews.

The research methodology "writing as inquiry" was described in 1994.

> Although we usually think about writing as a mode of "telling" about the social world, writing is not just a mopping-up activity at the end of a research project. Writing is also a way of "knowing"—a method of discovery and analysis. By writing in different ways, we discover new aspects of our topic and our relationship to it.[3]

Richardson goes on to explain that an author writes in order to find something out, to "learn something I didn't know before I wrote it."[4] We were taught in school not to write *until* we had something to say. This method of not writing *until* you have something to say "has serious problems: It ignores the role of writing as a dynamic, creative process."[5] However, with writing as inquiry, the writing propels the knowing, and as with Richardson, our own experience of inquiry was achieved in this poststructural nature.[6]

This search for insight about breastfeeding in the U.S. health care system also uses a research methodology described by Cooper, the integrative research review. An integrative research review appears independent of new data and is unlike a review of the literature.[7] "Integrative reviews summarize past research by drawing overall conclusions from many separate studies that are believed to address the state of knowledge concerning the relation(s) of interest and to highlight important issues that research has left unresolved."[8]

We also took into account the experiences of health care providers who have been successful at implementing breastfeeding strategies in their communities, strategies that are aimed at making breastfeeding a reality for women who choose to nurse their babies. In many ways, these people are alike. For example, they share a commitment to their work and their community. At the same time, they have a variety of professional backgrounds and personal experiences. We believe their knowledge is helpful, even inspirational, to others who want to reclaim breastfeeding in their communities.

A New Environment for Reclaiming Breastfeeding in the Health Care System

Unlike other Western industrialized nations, the United States does not have a policy of universal access to health care. In spite of unequal distribution of care, the U.S. per-capita cost of direct health care services is the highest in the world. As a percentage of gross national product (GNP), the U.S. also spends more than any other nation on health care with a rate of growth that is predicted to put expenditures at 15.9 percent of GNP by 2010 if the increase has not sufficiently been curbed.[9]

> Health expenditures increased 2,270 percent (between 1950 and 1990), with a marked increase in hospital usage. . . . [This] reflect[s] a serious misallocation of resources toward expensive medical practice. . . .[10]

Recognition of the exponentially increasing cost of health care, especially in the public sector through programs such as Medicare and Medicaid, prompted federal cost-cutting measures in 1983. A national program was phased in that reimbursed hospitals receiving Medicare payments *prospectively* by diagnosis rather than *retrospectively* for itemized services. This national system of payment became known as DRG, for Diagnostic Related Groups, reflecting the way payment was organized. Hospitals would now be paid a set fee for a person admitted who was a Medicare participant with a certain diagnosis. Payment under DRGs would be determined by the nature of the illness, not, as previously, by the quantity of services rendered. Payment in the old "fee-for-service" system was based on medical care, and each service was billed and reimbursed separately. Each provider in the system focused on the patient only in the setting in which they worked. The first effect of the change to DRGs was a dramatic Medicare-generated decrease in hospital income.[11] For the first time, health care providers and institutions had an economic incentive to reduce their costs.[12]

Increasing Quality to Decrease Costs

A phenomena that emerged in the health care sector after taking hold in the manufacturing industry was the idea that increased quality was one answer to the competition and financial pressures of cost reduction. The argument was put forward that higher quality health care would ultimately be reflected in the bottom line.[13] Hospitals and other providers that delivered higher-quality health care, it was believed, would be the survivors of the cutback in excess bed capacity that would result from the change to prospective reimbursement. Using DRGs would reduce length of hospital stays, so fewer beds would be needed.

New performance measures were needed, and in the late 1980s and early 1990s interest in customer satisfaction as a measure of quality increased.[14] Data collection from customers had resulted in improved services in industry[15] and so had the use of quality improvement processes. In 1989, Berwick, writing in the *New England Journal of Medicine,* suggested that the Continuous Quality Improvement systems (CQI) that were thought to be so effective in other businesses should become the new paradigm for health care.[16]

The third-party payment system in the United States gives payers strong and legitimate interest in the services provided. In the past two decades, payers have placed a growing emphasis on outcomes management[17] with performance-based capitated contracts for clinicians and institutions in the health care delivery arena. The routine communication of billing information enables the payer to aggregate information about patterns of care, to compare providers, and to use the information to contain costs.[18]

Other data sets have also been developed, and continue to be developed, to determine the outcomes of clinical care. The National Committee on Quality Assurance (NCOQA) and the Joint Commission on Accreditation and Healthcare Organizations (JCAHO) are two examples.

> . . . performance measurement dramatically changes the expectations of practice. Previously, a clinician's responsibility was to do everything possible for patients who took the initiative to visit the office. But achieving specific health outcomes means paying attention to patients who do not actively seek out care, and to factors, such as compliance and health seeking behaviors, that depend on more than what medical practitioners can do in their offices.[19]

None of the data sets track breastfeeding practices or services. In the public sector, the Healthy People objectives are reported and updated every 10 years, providing population-based goals for health. The Healthy People objectives have had breastfeeding initiation and duration goals for 1990, 2000, and 2010.

In the United States, the most consistently published information about breastfeeding incidence and duration is collected by a manufacturer of a brand of formula through the Ross Mothers' Survey. However, the federal government also uses a variety of methods to obtain data on breastfeeding incidence and duration. The Centers for Disease Control and Prevention (CDC) periodically collects statistics on breastfeeding through national surveys such as the National Survey of Family Growth, the National Health Interview Survey, the National Maternal and Infant Health Survey, and the National Health and Nutrition Examination Survey. In addition, breastfeeding statistics for many states are available through the Pregnancy Risk Assessment Monitoring System and the Pregnancy and Pediatric Nutrition Surveillance Systems. Additionally, the national standard birth certificate includes data on breastfeeding initiation. In 2001, CDC began collecting breastfeeding statistics on an ongoing basis for all states through the addition of questions to the National Immunization Survey. Through this survey, breastfeeding initiation and duration data will be available nationally every year and will be available for individual states and large metropolitan areas every 3–4 years.[20]

Systems theorists Senge and Asay have proposed a model to achieve "success" in the larger health care system, where success is defined as minimum cost and maximum reduction of disease symptoms. In this model, a successful program would maximize the number of healthy people, as well as maximize the speed and minimize the cost involved in returning people who need health care services and treatment to the healthy sector. In the old system, the "disease treatment" system, where success is defined only as moving people effectively and efficiently out of the "in-treatment" sector, the personal behaviors that cause people to need treatment occur outside the system. Senge and Asay's model of a successful health care system includes health and support of healthful-promoting personal behaviors, such as breastfeeding, *inside the health care system.*[21]

The term *managed care* represents an array of approaches in the organization of the delivery of health care, including health maintenance organizations (HMOs) and preferred provider organizations (PPOs). Managed-care programs may be for-profit or not-for-profit. The for-profit plans need to not only manage expenses to stay competitive, but also to distribute a financial return to their stockholders.

By 1994 two-thirds of all privately insured Americans were enrolled in an HMO or a PPO. One hundred million Americans were enrolled in managed-care health plans by 1998. The ideal managed-care system thoughtfully coordinates each member's health care, promotes preventive practices and behaviors such as breastfeeding, and monitors quality, thereby reducing costs. In the long run, the higher cost of treating illness would be replaced with the more efficient costs related to health promotion. The Conwal survey of the interaction between managed care and prevention resources indicates that the implementation of health-promotion activities within managed-care systems continues to be far from ideal.[22] As the managed-care industry incorporates and develops behavioral health promotion and health education, the focus of the medical community must change to improving and maintaining the health of the well, rather than primarily treating the not well. Breastfeeding, with its acknowledged health-promotion and prevention attributes, fits this new model.

Issues of Collaboration Between Medicine and Public Health

After World War II, the health system in the United States diverged into two distinct sectors: the "medical" sector and the "public health" sector. The medical sector perspective became that of health in regard to an individual patient; the public health sector focus became that of populations.

> To a large extent, tensions between the two sectors have been fueled by competition and concerns that public health—and the government in general—was infringing on physician autonomy and interfering with the doctor-patient relationship. . . . For example, threatened by public health efforts that might provide free services to patients by whom they might otherwise be paid, some physicians actively resisted well-baby clinics, health centers, and mass immunization programs.[23]

Managed care involves the assumption of financial risk by the provider because benefits are predetermined at a fixed price. In order to do this economically, it is not enough to control costs; providers must also anticipate health service demands accurately. Public health strategies are particularly well-suited to provide population-based data on health status and health risks. Under managed care, in striking contrast to fee-for-service or cost-based payments, treating medical problems consumes the medical sector's resources instead of increasing its revenues.[24]

Traditionally, the medical sector focused on "healers" who provided care for individuals when they were "sick," while the population-oriented public health sector focused on promoting healthful conditions for the community at large. The emphasis of medicine, then, was on healing individual illness, and the emphasis of public health was on population-based disease prevention. Over time, and with no economic incentives for the two sectors to collaborate, separate and independent health systems, contesting for limited resources, developed in the United States.

The changes in the health care system, restructuring according to the rules of the marketplace, and the redefinition of the government's role in public health have created an environment of growing interdependence between medicine and public health.

About the Chapters

The primary focus of this book is breastfeeding in the United States. Where applicable, comparisons will be made to breastfeeding attitudes, practices, and policies of other countries.

The twelve chapters in this book have been designed to enlarge upon specific issues related to the work done and the work still yet to be done in order to reclaim breastfeeding. Breastfeeding was the normal way to feed infants and young children for perhaps 100,000 generations. The attempt is now being made to reclaim what was lost in only three or four generations. An estimated cost savings of $3.6 billion per year for three childhood illnesses could be realized if we accomplish our national goals.[25]

Chapter 1: An International Policy Perspective on Breastfeeding in the United States looks at United States policy through an international lens and includes a chronology of major policy achievements in the past seven decades.

Chapter 2: Breastfeeding: A Public Health Policy Priority explores in depth the cornerstones of breastfeeding policy in the United States and the progress made toward implementing these policies. The irrefutable advantages of breastfeeding, our national goals and objectives, and the Innocenti Declaration are included.

Chapter 3: Using the Baby-Friendly Hospital Initiative to Drive Positive Change describes the implementation of the WHO/UNICEF Baby-Friendly Hospital Initiative (BFHI) in the United States, including a review of the relationship between the BFHI and improved breastfeeding outcomes.

Chapter 4: Breastfeeding, Quality, and the Health Care System explores the research related to breastfeeding initiation and duration and common hospital routines, such as rooming-in, early feedings, routine supplementation of the breastfed baby with formula, quality improvement projects, and the education of health care providers.

Chapter 5: Lactation Management: A Community of Practice proposes a work-study approach to evaluate the current state of practitioners who provide services as lactation workers, raising questions about the profession of lactation management worker.

Chapter 6: Toward Evidence-Based Breastfeeding Practice develops an evidence-based framework for evaluating interventions related to providing lactation care. An example is a review of the evidence base of the use of cabbage leaves to mitigate postpartum breast engorgement. (Portions of this Chapter have been adapted from the white paper of the same name previously published by Health Education Association).

Chapter 7: Defining Breastfeeding in Research examines definitions of breastfeeding and breastfeeding duration used in the 186 published research studies with a health outcome. The definitions of breastfeeding in studies in which at least one dependent outcome variable reached significance were compared to those used in studies in which no significance was found.

Chapter 8: Personal Motivations for Breastfeeding explores research findings related to how to best encourage mothers to choose between breastfeeding and formula feeding and how to support both the choice to breastfeed and the continuation of breastfeeding.

Chapter 9: Overcoming Disparities in Breastfeeding questions the reasons for the differences in the rates of breastfeeding initiation and duration among different groups of women. The chapter develops the concepts of peer counseling and cultural competency related to breastfeeding.

Chapter 10: Lactation and the Workplace reviews the literature related to reasons for the decrease in duration of breastfeeding observed for employed mothers and strategies designed to promote breastfeeding in employed mothers. Employer benefits that accrue with enhanced breastfeeding accommodation in the workplace are also reviewed.

Chapter 11: Human Milk for Fragile Infants examines human milk as a critical factor in the survival of fragile babies, including the human rights framework, hospital practices that affect breastfeeding of fragile babies, and the delivery of human milk.

Chapter 12: Using Banked Donor Milk in Clinical Settings describes the benefits and clinical uses of banked donor milk in the United States, including screening and processing. An international perspective is offered, as well as recommendations for the future.

References and Notes

1. Morse, J. 1994. Designing funded qualitative research. In *Handbook of Qualitative Research*. N. Denzin and Y. Lincoln, eds. Thousand Oaks: Sage Publications.
2. Richardson, L. 1994. Writing as inquiry. In *Handbook of Qualitative Research*. N. Denzin and Y. Lincoln, eds. Thousand Oaks: Sage Publications.

3. Richardson, L. 1994. Writing: A method of inquiry. In *Handbook of Qualitative Research,* N. Denzin and Y. Lincoln, eds., Thousand Oaks: Sage Publishers. 516.
4. Ibid.
5. Ibid., 517.
6. Poststructuralism reflects the belief that language and discourse produce meaning. "Understanding language as competing discourses, competing ways of giving meaning and of organizing the world, makes language a site of exploration, struggle." Ibid. 518.
7. Cooper. H. 1994. *The Integrative Research Approach.* Beverly Hills: Sage Publications.
8. Price, D. 1965. Networks of Scientific Papers. *Science.* 149: 510.
9. Thorpe, K. 1992. Health care cost containment: Results and lessons from the past 20 years. In *Improving Health Policy: Nine Critical Research Issues for the 1990s.* S. Shortell and U. Reinhardt, eds. Ann Arbor: Health Administration Press. 227.
   HCFA. 2001. National health expenditures projections: 2000–2010. *Health Affairs.* March/April. Accessed 9/1/2001 at http://www.healthaffairs.org.
10. Eastaugh, S. 1992. *Health Economics: Efficiency, Quality and Equity.* Westport, CT: Auburn House.
11. Ibid., 9.
12. Gray, B. 1991. *The Profit Motive and Patient Care.* Cambridge: Harvard University Press. 39.
13. Bewick, D. 1989. Continuous improvement as an ideal in health care. *NEJM.* 320(1), 53–55. Eastaugh, K. S. 1992. 233.
14. Leebov, W., and G. Scott. 1994. *Service Quality Improvement: The Customer Satisfaction Strategy for Health Care.* American Hospital Publishing, Inc. 3.
15. Schmidt, W., and J. Finnigan. 1992. *The Race without a Finish Line: America's Quest for Total Quality.* San Francisco: Jossey-Bass Publishers. 322.
16. Berwick, R. 1989. Continuous improvement as an ideal in health care. *NEJM* 320: 53–55.
17. Ellwood, P. 1988. Outcomes management: A technology of patient experience. *NEJM* 318: 1549–56.
18. Gray, B. H. 1991. *The Profit Motive and Patient Care: The Changing Accountability of Doctors and Hospitals.* Cambridge: Harvard University Press.
19. Lasker, R. D. 1997. *Medicine and Public Health: The Power of Collaboration.* New York: The New York Academy of Medicine. 41.
20. Grummer-Strawn, L. 2001. Personal Communication. September 26, 2001.
21. Senge, P., and D. Asay. 1988. Rethinking the Healthcare System. *Healthcare Forum Journal.* May/June: 32.
22. Stoil, M., and G. Hill. n.d. Interaction between managed care and prevention resources: A preliminary analysis of eight models. Conwal Incorporated. In press.

23. Lasker, R. D. 1997. *Medicine and Public Health: The Power of Collaboration*. New York: The New York Academy of Medicine. 17.

24. Ibid. 37.

25. Weimer, J. 2001. *The Economic Benefits of Breastfeeding: A Review and Analysis*. Food Assistance and Nutrition Research Report No. 13. Food and Economics Division, Economic Research Service, United States Department of Agriculture. Alexandria, VA: USDA.

ABOUT THE AUTHORS

Karin Cadwell, Ph.D., R.N., I.B.C.L.C., is a nationally and internationally recognized speaker, researcher, educator, and faculty member of the Healthy Children Project. She convened Baby-Friendly USA, implementing the UNICEF Baby-Friendly Hospital Initiative in the United States, was a visiting professor and program chair of the Health Communications Department of Emerson College, is a member of the United States Breastfeeding Committee, is a member of the Board of Directors of Healthy Mothers/Healthy Babies and former Chair of the National Healthy Mothers/Healthy Babies Breastfeeding Committee, and has led the Eisenhower Foundation annual international P.T.P. delegation on breastfeeding and human lactation exchanges to other nations. She is the author of numerous books and articles, was awarded the designation I.B.C.L.C. in 1985 for "significant contribution to the field" and has since recertified by exam.

Cindy Turner-Maffei, M.A., I.B.C.L.C., is national coordinator of Baby-Friendly USA, a faculty member of Healthy Children Project, and adjunct faculty of The Union Institute and University. She has extensive experience as a nutritionist and breastfeeding educator in W.I.C. and other Maternal Child Health programs. A member of breastfeeding coalitions on the local, state, and national level, including the Massachusetts Breastfeeding Committee and the United States Breastfeeding Committee, she is also an author and editor of *The Curriculum to Support the Ten Steps to Successful Breastfeeding* and *Maternal and Infant Assessment for Breastfeeding and Human Lactation.*

Anna Blair, Ph.D., is a researcher and faculty member of the Healthy Children Project. Dr. Blair's work has included research on sore nipples and positioning/latch. She is an adjunct faculty of the Union Institute and University/Healthy Children Maternal and Child Health: Lactation Consulting degree. She is a co-author of *Maternal and Infant Assessment for Breastfeeding and Human Lactation*. She counsels breastfeeding mothers on Cape Cod, Mass., who have given birth prematurely.

Lois D. W. Arnold, M.P.H., I.B.C.L.C., is the C.E.O. of the National Commission on Donor Milk Banking, an administrative consultant for Baby-Friendly U.S.A., and was the Executive Director of the Human Milk Banking Association of North America, Inc. for nine years. She is the author of numerous journal articles, the Independent Study Module Program Coordinator for La Leche League International, and a member of the United States Breastfeeding Committee. She has taught workshops, lectured at various conferences, and first became an I.B.C.L.C. in 1985.

Zoë Maja McInerney, M.A., C.L.C., is a doctoral candidate at the University of Connecticut in Industrial/Organizational Psychology. Her research focus has been work-family conflict and balance. Zoë also works as a researcher and data analyst at the Institute for Community Inclusion at Children's Hospital in Boston. The I.C.I.'s research focuses on the multiple influences affecting the quality of life for people with disabilities, including personal supports and relationships, professional support strategies, organizational influences, and state and federal policy.

Charles M. Cadwell, Ph.D., has advanced degrees in mathematics and research methods in behavioral medicine. He is a research consultant for the Healthy Children Project and the production head of Health Education Associates.

Kajsa Brimdyr, Ph.D., works primarily in the field of People, Computers and Work and teaches at the Blekinge Institute of Technology in southern Sweden. She consults with the Healthy Children Project's Center for Breastfeeding regarding educational programs in Health Education.

CHAPTER ONE

AN INTERNATIONAL POLICY PERSPECTIVE ON BREASTFEEDING IN THE UNITED STATES

Karin Cadwell, Ph.D., R.N., I.B.C.L.C.

Promoting, Protecting, and Supporting Breastfeeding

We have lost breastfeeding as the cultural norm in the United States. An excellent model for understanding modern issues about breastfeeding can be found in the title of a 1989 publication of the World Health Organization (WHO) and UNICEF: *Protecting, Promoting and Supporting Breastfeeding.*

Breastfeeding **promotion** efforts focus on the advantages of breastfeeding as they apply to the individual baby and mother. "Promotion efforts" also include the communication of the many advantages of breastfeeding in regard to the global ecology: decreased waste from bottles and the manufacturing process, the diminished environmental cost of the care and feeding of dairy cattle, and resulting decrease in methane in the environment.

Breastfeeding **protection** involves the legislated rights of women and children that serve to enable breastfeeding. These rights include adequate maternity leaves, appropriate child care facilities, and nursing breaks for women in the workplace. Protection of breastfeeding also involves prohibiting certain marketing practices of companies that manufacture breast milk substitutes and includes the prohibition of free samples of infant foods and direct advertising of these commodities to consumers.

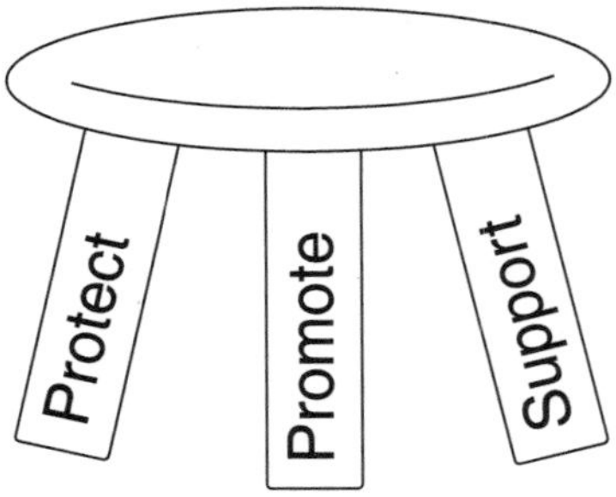

FIGURE 1.1   Successful
breastfeeding stool.

Breastfeeding **support** is accomplished through evidenced-based hospital policies and health provider practices and community programs, such as peer counselors and mother-to-mother support, that serve to increase breastfeeding initiation, exclusivity, and duration.

Promoting, protecting, and supporting have been described as three legs of a breastfeeding stool as shown in Figure 1.1. In order to reclaim breastfeeding in our bottle-feeding culture, all three legs are necessary, or the stool—successful breastfeeding—will not stand.

> "Breastfeeding is an endangered practice. It needs an entire culture to support and nurture it back to its full, patent strength." (UNICEF)

Even before World War II had started, some European physicians began to see that breastfeeding was threatened by the aggressive marketing practices of infant formula companies. They began to recommend that breastfeeding be protected. As these visionaries could foresee, traditional, "unprotected" breastfeeding was endangered but could be protected if a society chose to do so. A UNICEF publication entitled *Take the Baby-Friendly Initiative* summarizes the issue.[1]

We know that when a species is endangered, protection is needed. When whales were abundant, they did not need to be protected (or promoted or supported). Now whales do need protection, as do many other endangered species. Even after breastfeeding becomes the cultural norm, protection will continue to be important.

Some countries have recognized that breastfeeding needs to be protected and they have made social changes and moved to protect breastfeeding through legal means. In a fairly short period of time, Sweden, for example, nearly countrywide, has brought back almost universal breastfeeding. In 1973, in both Sweden and the United States, most babies were formula fed and only about 20 percent of newborn babies were breastfed.[2]

By 1988, Sweden had an 85 percent initiation rate. The United States had achieved an initiation rate of 55 percent during the same time period. The differences are more notable for slightly older babies. The Swedes looked at breastfeeding among four-month-old infants in

1992 and found that 75 percent of the babies were still being breast-fed. Only about 20 percent of U.S. babies were breastfed at 5–6 months of age in 1992. Indeed, the exclusive breastfeeding rates in the United States have been in an overall pattern of decline since 1983–1984[3]. Many babies receive supplemental formula in the hospital, even before breastfeeding has begun for the mother who intends to breastfeed. Figure 1.2 shows a significant decline in exclusive breastfeeding between 1990 and 1998.

According to a 1994 study in Denmark, breastfeeding rates were high, with 99.5 percent of mothers initiating breastfeeding. In babies' first three months, 71 percent of mothers were still breastfeeding; in six months, 52 percent, and in nine months, 33 percent. Formula supplements given during the first days of life to some babies were associated with shorter duration of breastfeeding, and "the difference was substantial."[4] An important part of the Baby-Friendly Hospital Initiative is avoiding formula supplements given for non-medical reasons. For example, breastfeeding rates in Denmark were considerably higher in the 1990s than in the late 1970s. In the later period 52 percent of mothers of six-month-old babies were still nursing, as compared to 25–30 percent in the earlier period.

It is still popular and politically correct in the United States to put the blame for the decline in breastfeeding on mothers' return to the workforce, although a number of studies disagree.[5,6,7,8,9] In a 1998 study, the breastfeeding of mothers who expected to work full time was found to differ significantly from that of mothers who expected to work part time. Part-time work was found to be an effective strategy to help

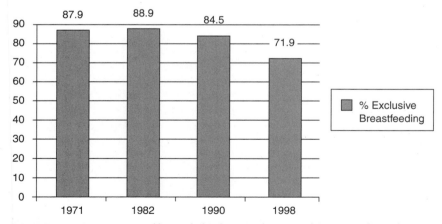

FIGURE 1.2   Percentages of breastfed infants in the United States exclusively breastfeeding at hospital discharge.
Source: Calculated using data from Ross Mothers' Survey, Ross Products Division, Abbott Laboratories.

FIGURE 1.3 Lopsided
breastfeeding stool.

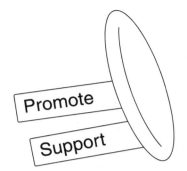

mothers combine breastfeeding and employment. Part-time was defined as fewer than thirty-five hours per week, or a maximum of seven
hours per day.[10] Mothers gave up breastfeeding in the early days because they were afraid that they did not have enough milk, not because
they might return to work a few weeks later.

Breastfeeding is not the cultural norm in the United States for many
reasons. One of the reasons is that we have a lopsided stool, one lack-
ing a protective leg (Figure 1.3).

Once breastfeeding has become endangered, it needs consistent
promotion, support, and protection. The UNICEF Baby-Friendly Hospital Initiative protects mothers in maternity facilities from products that
promote formula. When Dr. Natividad Reclucio-Clavano threw infant
formula representatives out of a hospital nursery in the Philippines, she
was "protecting" breastfeeding as well as supporting and promoting it.

> I closed the door of the nursery to the milk companies. We stopped
> giving our babies the starter dose of infant formula. Down came the
> colorful posters and calendars; in their place we hung "baby killer"
> posters which show an emaciated baby inside a dirty feeding bottle.
> Would the milk companies sue me? I wondered. Everything that was
> conducive to bottle–feeding was removed not only from the nursery,
> but from everywhere in the hospital. I myself rejected samples and
> donations from the milk companies. How else could we be credible?[11]

The Politics of Breastfeeding

We need to identify what we have accomplished in our efforts to reclaim breastfeeding so that we might better understand how to move
forward in the future. In order to be able to clearly understand the recent history of breastfeeding promotion, protection, and support, the
chronology in Table 1.1 has been constructed.

TABLE 1.1   Chronology of Breastfeeding History

1939	Dr. Cicely Williams publishes the book *Milk and Murder.* In a speech to the Singapore Rotary Club, Dr. Williams says that "misguided propaganda on infant feeding" should be considered "murder." Dr. Williams seems to have been the first authority to point out that breastfeeding in the modern world needed protection.
1956	La Leche League is started by nursing mothers who met for a picnic in a suburb of Chicago. As they discussed their own difficulties in nursing their first babies, they realized that new mothers needed encouragement and advice from experienced breastfeeders. La Leche, started as a small grass roots support group, has experienced enormous growth and has thousands of leaders in all fifty states and in many other nations.
1968	Dr. Derrick Jelliffe in Jamaica coins the term "commerciogenic malnutrition" to describe the impact of the baby food/formula industry marketing practices on infant health.
1970	The United Nations Protein-Calorie Advisory Group (PAG) raises concern about the baby food/formula industry practices.
1972	International Organization of Consumers Union (IOCU) submits a draft code of practice on the advertising of infant foods to FAO/WHO Codex Alimentarius Commission.
1973	*New Internationalist* magazine publishes a cover story on the "Baby Food Tragedy." It calls for an action campaign to halt unethical promotion of baby milks. The United Nations PAG states that promotion of formula feeding to mothers in the hospital immediately after birth is inappropriate. War on Want publishes *The Baby Killer,* a report on infant malnutrition and the promotion of artificial feeding in the Third World. Berne Third World Action Group (AgDW) translates *The Baby Killer* and publishes it in Switzerland with the title *Nestlé Totet Babies* (Nestlé Kills Babies). Nestlé sues AgDW for libel. World Health Assembly recommends regulating inappropriate sales promotion of infant foods that replace breast milk.
1974	Women, Infants and Children (WIC) Program is authorized by the U.S. Congress. Low-income families receive free infant formula plus nutritional counseling. Its focus is to promote breastfeeding.
1976	A Swiss court warns Nestlé to change its marketing practices. This is the result of a lawsuit by Nestlé against campaigners who accused the company of killing babies. The Nestlé boycott begins. The American Academy of Pediatrics publishes a statement to promote breastfeeding. A major breastfeeding conference is held in Washington, DC. It is cosponsored by George Washington University, the March of Dimes, and the U.S. Public Health Service. U.S. nuns sue Bristol-Myers. Sisters of the Precious Blood file a lawsuit to draw attention to the threat to infant health caused by Nestlé's promotion of baby milk.
1977	Papua, New Guinea, bans advertisements for feeding bottles and requires prescriptions for bottles and teats. This is a successful effort to protect breastfeeding. INFACT launches Nestlé boycott in the U.S. to protest Nestlé's unethical marketing practices.

(continued)

TABLE 1.1 Chronology of Breastfeeding History *(continued)*

1978   The U.S. Senate conducts a hearing on the inappropriate marketing of baby milks in developing countries. It is seen as an issue for Third World countries, where protection against the formula companies is seen as necessary.

          The American Academy of Pediatrics issues a major commentary in support of breastfeeding for all full-term newborn infants. It recommends interventions that would support breastfeeding, such as rooming-in.

1979   World Health Organization (WHO) and UNICEF host an international meeting on infant and young child feeding. The meeting calls for the development of an international code of marketing as well as action on other fronts to improve infant and young child feeding practices.

          The International Baby Food Action Network (IBFAN) is founded.

1980   The Nestlé boycott is launched in the United Kingdom by Baby Milk Action (BMAC).

          The infant formula industry retracts its breastfeeding promotion pledge. In testimony at a United States Senate Hearing, Nestlé and three U.S. companies admit they do not intend to abide by World Health Organization's interpretation of the October 1979 WHO/UNICEF meeting.

1981   The International Code of Marketing of Breast-Milk Substitutes is adopted at the World Health Assembly. The "WHO Code" is passed by 118 votes to one, with only the U.S. voting against it. President Reagan's representative is persuaded to vote "no" by industry representatives. The Ambulatory Pediatric Association urges the United States delegate to vote for the Code and calls for an end to free formula distribution in hospitals. It is a major statement about protecting and supporting breastfeeding.

          The WHO Code of 1981 is considered a minimum requirement to protect breastfeeding. The WHO Code included:

- warnings of health hazards on labels of breast milk substitutes
- prohibition of free formula in the health care system
- prohibition of promotion of formula in any health care facilities
- prohibition of money or gifts to health workers
- required disclosure of industry contributions to conferences, research, etc.
- admonishing of governments to pass laws to implement the Code (Appendix B).

          The European Parliament votes for a directive based on the International Code.

          The Nestlé boycott is started in Sweden and the Federal Republic of Germany.

1982   Peru becomes the first country to adopt the International Code as national legislation. This law will protect breastfeeding from formula companies.

          A Nestlé boycott starts in France.

          The American Academy of Pediatrics issues a statement, The Promotion of Breastfeeding, stating that "educational materials should be factual and designed to present the advantage of breastfeeding but should not promote guilt among non-breastfeeding families."

1983   The European Parliament again passes a strongly worded resolution in favor of the WHO Code.

          The United Kingdom introduces a voluntary code, based on proposals from the Food Manufacturers Federation (FMF), despite strong criticism from health worker bodies and action groups who consider it weak.

          The Nestlé boycott spreads to Norway and Finland. The boycott in North America intensifies.

1984　Nestlé agrees to implement the International Code. Boycott groups agree to suspend the boycott for six months in order to allow Nestlé time to put its promises into practice.

The first Nestlé boycott ends.

The World Health Assembly (WHA) adopts a resolution cautioning against using formula and other manufactured infant foods in early infancy.

United States Surgeon General C. Everett Koop convenes the Surgeon General's Workshop on Breastfeeding and Human Lactation. Recommendations are made by work groups:

- Category 1: World of Work—A national breastfeeding promotion initiative, directed to all those who influence the breastfeeding decisions and opportunities of women involved in school, job training, professional education, and employment, is needed.
- Category 2: Public Education—Public education and promotion efforts should be undertaken through the educational system and the media. Such efforts should recognize the diversity of the audience; should target various economic, cultural, and ethnic groups; and should be coordinated with professional education.
- Category 3: Professional Education—It is imperative to receive adequate didactic and clinical training in lactation and breastfeeding and to develop skills in patient education and the management of breastfeeding.

1985　IBFAN launches a series of regular training workshops in Africa and publishes the first edition of *Protecting Infant Health,* which is a health worker's guide to the WHO Code.

WHO/UNICEF Committee of Experts calls for an end to free supplies of formula.

1986　The World Health Assembly passes a resolution banning free and subsidized supplies of infant formula.

The European Parliament votes to include most of the provisions of the WHO Code in its draft direction.

1988　The United States group Action (formerly INFACT) boycotts Nestlé and Wyeth/American Home Products (AHP) because of free supplies to hospitals in developing nations.

1989　The United Kingdom announces it will ban free and low-cost formula and feeding supplies effective January 1, 1989.

The General Assembly in the United Nations holds a convention on Rights of the Child.

Boycotts of Nestlé are launched in the United Kingdom, Ireland, Norway, and Sweden.

WHO/UNICEF publish "Protecting, Promoting and Supporting Breastfeeding." The three components are recognized as essential to breastfeeding policy.

The WIC reauthorization requires the states to spend a designated portion of nutrition service funding on breastfeeding promotion. The General Accounting Office (GAO) publishes a report entitled "Breastfeeding: WIC's Efforts to Promote Breastfeeding Have Increased."

1990　The Innocenti Declaration on the Protection, Promotion and Support of Breastfeeding is adopted by health policy makers from government and United Nations agencies, including the United States. It calls on all governments to implement the WHO Code by 1995. This international document calls for specific goals for 1995, including:

- appoint a national breastfeeding coordinator,
- enact legislation protection for the breastfeeding rights of working women,
- take action to give effect to the WHO Code and other World Health Assembly resolutions, and
- ensure that all maternity facilities practice Ten Steps to Successful Breastfeeding from "Protecting, Promoting and Supporting Breastfeeding: The Special Role of Maternity Services" (WHO/UNICEF).

(continued)

TABLE 1.1   Chronology of Breastfeeding History   *(continued)*

The Ten Steps would receive much attention, as they are to be the focus of the Baby-Friendly Hospital Initiative.

In the Healthy People 2000 objectives, the U.S. Secretary of Health and Human Services sets goals for breastfeeding. The goals are to "increase at least 75 percent of the proportion of mothers who breastfeed their babies in the early postpartum period and at least 50 percent of the proportion who continue breastfeeding until their babies are five to six months old."

1992   U.S. Federal Trade Commission charges infant formula companies with bid-rigging in the WIC program. (Formula will continue to be given to low-income families but should be purchased as inexpensively as possible.)

An "expert work group" is convened to conduct "a Feasibility Study of the Implementation of the Baby-Friendly Hospital Initiative in the United States." Healthy Mothers/Healthy Babies (HMHB) is funded to conduct a three-year study.

UNICEF and WHO, at World Summit for Children, launch the Baby-Friendly Hospital Initiative as a worldwide movement. One goal created to protect breastfeeding continues.

The first annual World Breastfeeding Week is celebrated.

1993   The *Wall Street Journal* publishes an article entitled "Spilt Milk: Methods of Marketing Infant Formula Land Abbot in Hot Water."

Bristol-Myers Squibb (the parent company of Mead Johnson) and American Home Products Corporation (the parent company of Wyeth-Ayerst) settle with the Florida Attorney General, agreeing to pay the state $5 million in response to allegations of price-fixing and conspiracy to drive up the cost of formula through a marketing scheme that eliminated direct advertising. Abbot Laboratories (parent to Ross Products Division) settles just hours before the trial is to begin, according to the "WIC Newsletter" (June 24, 1993). This story also highlighted the relationship between the major formula manufacturers and the American Academy of Pediatrics (AAP) and reported that the formula manufacturers contribute substantially each year to the AAP.

UNICEF seeks to empower all women in industrialized countries to breastfeed exclusively.

1994   The World Health Assembly passes a Resolution (WHA Resolution 47.5) which supports the WHO Code.

President Clinton signs WHA Resolution 47.5; thus the United States agrees to the WHO Code, 13 years after the other 118 nations. This resolution specifies that no free or low-cost supplies of breast milk substitutes are allowed in any aspect of the health care system. It reinforces points from the 1981 Code and adds additional points. However, there is no legislative follow-up.

Just before World Breastfeeding Week, the *Wall Street Journal* publishes an article about breastfeeding, "Dying for Milk: Some Mothers Trying in Vain to Breastfeed, Starve Their Infants."

Reauthorization of WIC boosts breastfeeding promotion efforts and requires standardizing the collection of data on breastfeeding rates for infants enrolled in the program.

Results of the three-year Feasibility Study of Implementation of the Baby-Friendly Hospital Initiative in the United States are announced. Some members of the Expert Work Group submit letters in which they explain their minority positions.

1995	The USDA and Food and Consumer Service develops a WIC National Breast-feeding Promotion Project in a cooperative agreement with Best Start Social Marketing.
1996	The first hospital in the United States to be designated as a Baby-Friendly Hospital is announced. (There are more than 10,000 worldwide.) The announcement is made by Wellstart International and the U.S. Committee for UNICEF.
1997	The Healthy Children Project, a nonprofit research and educational institution, is asked by the U.S. Committee for UNICEF to found an independent non-profit, Baby-Friendly USA in order to implement the Baby-Friendly Hospital Initiative in the United States.
	The American Academy of Pediatrics, Work Group on Breastfeeding, publishes a statement "Breastfeeding and the Use of Human Milk," which summarizes "the benefits of breastfeeding to the infant, the mother, and the nation and sets forth principles to guide the pediatrician and other care providers in the initiation and maintenance of breastfeeding."
1998	The United States Breastfeeding Committee is established. This multisectoral national committee is called for in the first operational target of the Innocenti Declaration.
	The Barcello conference on National Breastfeeding Policy is held in Washington, DC. It is organized by the UCLA Center of Healthier Children, Families and Communities Breastfeeding Resource Program in cooperation with the U.S. Department of Health and Human Services Maternal and Child Health Bureau and others.
1999	Legislation is passed allowing women to breastfeed anywhere on U.S. government property where they are otherwise allowed to be.
	The United States "Curriculum to Support the Ten Steps to Successful Breastfeeding" is developed with funding from the U.S. Department of Health and Human Services, Public Health Service, Health Resources and Services Administration, Maternal & Child Health Bureau, and the Healthy Children 2000 Project.
	The Centers for Disease Control and Prevention (CDC) convenes a meeting of approximately thirty experts in breastfeeding and epidemiology in November to achieve a better understanding of how the breastfeeding status of children in the United States can be monitored through breastfeeding surveillance systems.
2000	The U.S. Strategic Plan for Breastfeeding, developed by the United States breastfeeding Committee, is completed.
	The Healthy People 2010 Objectives are announced. Along with the other target percentages of mothers who breastfeed, the breastfeeding objective includes a twelve- months goal for the first time:

Goal at initiation (early postpartum) 75%
Goal at six months   50%
Goal at twelve months   25%

	The Office on Women's Health of the U.S. Department of Health and Human Services releases the Health and Human Services Blueprint for Action on Breastfeeding,"[12] with a message from the Surgeon General, David Satcher, M.D., Ph.D., stating, "together we can shape a future in which mothers can feel comfortable and free to breastfeed their children without societal hinderances."[13]
2001	The United States Breastfeeding Committee releases its strategic plan "Breastfeeding in the United States: A National Agenda."[14] It describes four goals.
	Goal I: Assure access to comprehensive, current, and culturally appropriate lactation care and services for all women, children, and families.

(continued)

TABLE 1.1   Chronology of Breastfeeding History   *(concluded)*

Goal II: Ensure that breastfeeding is recognized as the normal and preferred method of feeding infants and young children.

Goal III: Ensure that all federal, state, and local laws relating to child welfare and family law recognize and support the importance and practice of breastfeeding.

Goal IV: Increase protection, promotion, and support for breastfeeding mothers in the workforce.

Baby-Friendly USA announces the thirty-second hospital to receive the Baby-Friendly designation in the United States.

References

1. UNICEF. 1992. *Take the Baby-Friendly Initiative.* New York: UNICEF.
2. Zetterstorm, R. 1994. Trends in research on infant nutrition, past, present and future. *Acta. Paediatr. Suppl.* 402:1.
3. Ross Laboratories. 1990. As reported by Office of Maternal and Child Health, Public Health Service, U.S. Department of Health and Human Services.
4. Michaelson, K. F. 1994. The Copenhagen cohort study on infant nutrition and growth: Duration of breastfeeding and influencing factors. *Acta. Paediatr.* 83:565.
5. Arafat, I. et al. 1981. Maternal practice and attitudes toward breastfeeding. *JOGN Nurs.* 10(2):91.
6. Gielen, A. 1991. Maternal employment during early postpartum period: Effects on initiation and constitution of breastfeeding. *Peds.* 87:298.
7. Hawkins, L. M. 1987. Predictors of the duration of breastfeeding in low-income women. *Birth* 14(4):204.
8. Laughlin, H. H. 1985. Early termination of breastfeeding: Identifying those at risk. *Peds.* 75(3):508.
9. Skinner, J. et al. 1997. Transition in infant feeding during the first year of life. *J. Am. Col. Nutr.* 16:3, 209.
10. Fein, S. B. et al. 1998. The effect of work status on initiation and duration of breastfeeding. *Am. J. Public Health* 88:1042.
11. Reclucio-Clavano, N. 1981. The results of a change in hospital practices: A pediatrician's campaign for breastfeeding in the Philippines. Assignment 55/56:139.
12. United States Department of Health and Human Services. 2000. "Health and Human Services Blueprint for Action on Breastfeeding," Washington DC: U.S. Department of Health and Human Services, Office on Women's Health.
13. United States Breastfeeding Committee. 2001. *Breastfeeding in the United States: A National Agenda.* Rockville, MD: U.S. Department of Health and Human Services, Health Resources and Services Administration, Maternal and Child Health Bureau.

CHAPTER TWO

BREASTFEEDING: A PUBLIC HEALTH POLICY PRIORITY

Karin Cadwell, Ph.D., R.N., I.B.C.L.C.

Breastfeeding is readily acknowledged to be the optimal way to nourish and nurture infants, and with the addition of complementary foods in the second half of the first year, it continues to be of nutritional, immunological, and psychological significance well into the second year and beyond. Statements in support of breastfeeding have been issued by professional associations and even Pope John Paul II.

Advantages of Breastfeeding for Recipient Infants and Young Children

The health advantages of breastfeeding for the recipient infant in an industrialized nation such as the United States have been described in multiple peer-reviewed, published medical research studies.[1] These advantages impact each of the following areas:

- Gastrointestinal illness: At least 400 infants die annually in the U.S. from diarrheal disease. An estimated 250–300 of these have been attributed to not being breastfed.[2] Other gastrointestinal problems such as Crohn's disease, inflammatory bowel disease, and celiac disease have been known to be minimized or diagnosed at a later age in people who have been breastfed.[3]
- Respiratory illness: The risk of fatal or nonfatal respiratory infections is two- to fivefold among nonbreastfed infants.[4]

11

- Otitis media: Occurs more frequently in infants who are not breast-fed or who are breastfed for shorter durations. The morbidity, inconvenience, and expense of ear infections is considerable.[5]
- Bacteremia and meningitis: The risk of these conditions is fourfold in babies who are not breastfed.[6]
- Juvenile diabetes: As many as 25 percent of cases of juvenile diabetes can be attributed to not being breastfed or to exposure to formula in infancy.[7]
- Malignant lymphomas in children: A six- to eightfold risk has been reported for the development of lymphomas in children under the age of fifteen who were not breastfed for six months.[8]
- Breast cancer: Women who were breastfed as children may have reduced breast cancer rates when over forty years of age by more than 25 percent.[9,10]
- Multiple sclerosis: Adults with multiple sclerosis were found to have been breastfed four months fewer than matched controls.[11]
- Allergies: Breastfeeding may delay the onset of allergic symptoms and decrease wheezing.[12]
- Other health problems: Other possible health problems associated with not being breastfed include decreased obesity[13], chronic respiratory disease, coronary artery disease, higher cholesterol in young adulthood, and ischemic heart disease.[4]

Psychomotor advantages of breastfeeding also have been described in multiple research studies published in peer-reviewed journals. They include:

- Breastfeeding has been found to mitigate the intellectual deficits in congenital cretinism.[14]
- In middle-income families, cognitive and motor development test scores increase in proportion to the increased duration of breast-feeding in infancy.[15]
- In premature infants who received their mother's milk for their early feeds, long-term follow-up shows a significant IQ advantage.[16]
- Visual acuity is less in children who received no breast milk or who received breast milk for a brief period of time.[17]
- Neuromotor skills in neurologically impaired children are measurably better in those who received breast milk.[18]

Advantages of Breastfeeding for Women Who Breastfeed

The health advantages for women who chose to breastfeed also have been described in peer-reviewed medical journals. They include:

- less postpartum bleeding and more rapid uterine involution
- less menstrual blood loss during the months after delivery
- earlier return to prepregnant weight[19]
- delayed resumption of ovulation, leading to longer child spacing
- improved bone remineralization in the postpartum[20] period
- reduction in hip fractures in the postmenopausal period[21]
- reduced risk of ovarian cancer
- reduced risk of premenopausal breast cancer

Social and Economic Benefits of Increased Breastfeeding

The social and economic benefits of breastfeeding have been estimated for only a fraction of the known health advantages and include:

- reduced health care costs
- reduced employee absenteeism for the care of ill infants
- reduced direct cost of breastfeeding in comparison to formula purchase
- reduced waste and environmental pollution

"Although knowledge about the benefits of breastfeeding appear to have been well disseminated to mothers and to health care professionals, the translation of that knowledge into behavior lags behind."[22]

The 1990 Breastfeeding Objectives

In 1984, C. Everett Koop convened the **Surgeon General's Workshop on Breastfeeding and Human Lactation.** The workshop served to review past efforts that had been made in the public and private sectors to promote breastfeeding, to assess challenges, and to "develop strategies and recommendations in order to facilitate progress toward achieving the 1990 objective"[23] of 75 percent of women breastfeed at hospital discharge and 35 percent nursing at six months of age.[24]

The recommendations generated at the workshop included:

- Improve professional education in human lactation and breastfeeding.
- Develop public education and promotional efforts.
- Strengthen the support for breastfeeding in the health care system.
- Develop a broad range of support services in the community.
- Initiate a national breastfeeding promotion effort directed to women in the workforce.
- Expand research in human lactation and breastfeeding.[23]

The second follow-up report to the Surgeon General's Workshop, published in 1991, reviewed the national, state and local efforts that had been initiated to attain these recommendations.[25]In spite of the many efforts enumerated in the follow-up report, early infancy breast-feeding rates increased fewer than 10 percentage points in the 1980s, as reflected in Figure 2.1. The rate of 54 percent in 1988 compared to 45.1 percent in 1978 repsents a deficit of 21 percentage points from the 1990 goal.[26]

The 1990 duration goal for breastfeeding was that 35 percent of women would continue to breastfeed their babies five to six months of age. In 1971 only 5.5 percent of women breastfed their babies at five to six months of age. The baseline number for the 1990 goals was 20.5 percent, but by 1988 there had been no significant increase in duration. As shown in Figure 2.2, only 21 percent of women continued to breast-feed their babies at five to six months of age.

Unlike the 1990 Goals for the Nation that were developed within the federal government, the leadership for the process of developing health objectives for the year 2000 came from "every level of government—national, state and local—from professional groups, and from multiple sectors of American communities working through a Healthy People 2000 Consortium of more than 300 organizations."[27]

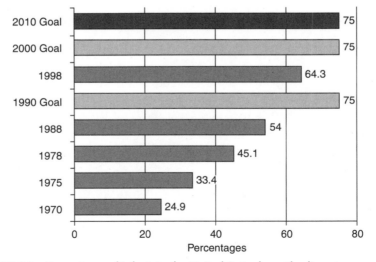

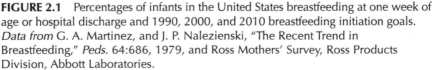

FIGURE 2.1 Percentages of infants in the United States breastfeeding at one week of age or hospital discharge and 1990, 2000, and 2010 breastfeeding initiation goals. *Data from* G. A. Martinez, and J. P. Nalezienski, "The Recent Trend in Breastfeeding," *Peds.* 64:686, 1979, and Ross Mothers' Survey, Ross Products Division, Abbott Laboratories.

The **Healthy People 2000** objective for breastfeeding was to "increase to at least 75 percent the proportion of mothers who breastfed their babies in the early postpartum period and to at least 50 percent the proportion who continue breastfeeding until their babies are 5 to 6 months old."[28] The in-hospital breastfeeding rate for 1998 was 64.3 percent[29] substantially lower than the 75 percent year 2000 objective and an increase of only 10.3 percentage points over the 1988 baseline. In 1998 only 28.6 percent were reported continuing to six months, an increase of only 7.6 percentage points from 1988 and 8.1 percent from 1978 (See Figures 2.1 and 2.2).

The baseline data used was from the 1988 Ross Laboratories Mothers' Survey with special target population collected by the Pediatric Nutrition Surveillance System, Centers for Disease Control (CDC). Although special population targets such as African American mothers, Hispanic mothers, and American Indian/Alaska Native mothers were identified, the 2000 goal of 75 percent breastfeeding initiation with 50 percent continuing at five to six months was the same for all population groups.

In December 1990 the Maternal Child Health Bureau (MCHB) and the U.S. Department of Health and Human Services (DHHS) held a national workshop, **Call to Action: Better Nutrition for Mothers, Children, and Families.** This forum, held in Washington, DC, was structured

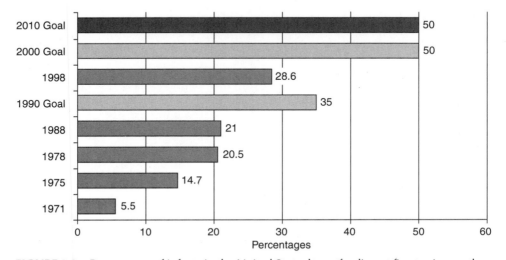

FIGURE 2.2 Percentages of infants in the United States breastfeeding at five to six months of age and 1990, 2000, and 2010 breastfeeding objective for five to six months of age. Data from G. A. Martinez and J. P. Nalezienski, "The Recent Trend in Breastfeeding," *Peds.* 64:691, 1979, and Ross Mothers' Survey, Ross Products Divisible Abbott Laboratories.

on "identifying current needs and issues in maternal and child nutrition services, reaching a consensus on priorities, developing key recommendations, and outlining specific actions and strategies which should be taken to implement the recommendations."[30] A collaborative approach to problem solving and program development among agencies and organizations was emphasized.

Recommendation 8 of the Call to Action became "to promote breastfeeding among all women to achieve the year 2000 National Health Promotion and Disease Prevention Objectives for breastfeeding, and establish breastfeeding as the societal norm for infant feeding." Strategies for achieving the year 2000 objectives for breastfeeding were:

1. Promote breastfeeding as the preferred method of infant feeding to the memberships of all health professional organizations.
2. Continue efforts to develop more effective strategies to promote breastfeeding through hospitals, MCH programs, WIC and other food assistance programs, industry, and other worksites, including federal agencies.
3. Explore ways to promote breastfeeding through community programs, such as the EFNEP, food stamps, and other community-based interventions.
4. Encourage federal agencies to serve as models for providing support of breastfeeding women in the federal worksite.
5. Assure that health care professionals who interact with pregnant women, including hospital personnel, communicate breastfeeding as the norm.
6. Continue to develop and implement ways to support and provide incentives for breastfeeding in the WIC program.
7. Include specific methods of supporting breastfeeding in the standards of practice for health professionals.
8. Provide lactation management training to all health care professionals who interact with pregnant and breastfeeding women to enhance their ability to support breastfeeding, and involve hospitals in networking for the promotion of breastfeeding.[31]

Call to Action recommendations 12, 13, and 14 also addressed breastfeeding concerns such as the marketing of infant foods and formula to consumers, the need for reliable and standardized data on infant feeding practices, and research priorities in the area of infant nutrition. Because the Call to Action was collaborative and included organizations with an interest in promoting breastfeeding, these recommendations were intended to be implemented in both the public and private sectors.

The Innocenti Declaration on the Protection, Promotion, and Support of Breastfeeding was produced and adopted in 1990 in Spedale degli Innocenti, Florence, Italy. The meeting, Breastfeeding in the 1990s: A Global Initiative, was cosponsored by the United States

Agency for International Development (USAID) and the Swedish International Development Authority (SIDA). The Declaration, adopted by participants, including the United States, at the WHO/UNICEF policy makers meeting included four operational targets. All governments by the year 1995 should have:

1. appointed a national breastfeeding coordinator of appropriate authority and established a multisectoral national breastfeeding committee composed of representatives from relevant government departments, nongovernmental organizations, and health professional associations;
2. ensured that every facility providing maternity services fully practices all ten of the Ten Steps to Successful Breastfeeding set out in the joint WHO/UNICEF statement Protecting, Promoting and Supporting Breast-Feeding: The Special Role of Maternity Services;
3. taken action to give effect to the principles and aim of all Articles of the International Code of Marketing of Breast-Milk Substitutes and subsequent relevant World Health Assembly resolutions in their entirety; and
4. enacted imaginative legislation protecting the breastfeeding rights of working women and established means for its enforcement.[32]

In regard to the operational targets that were generated from the Innocenti Declaration, the United States established a multisectoral national breastfeeding committee in Orlando, Florida, on January 19, 1998, called for in the first operational target. A breastfeeding coordinator of appropriate authority had not been appointed by the end of 2001. The National Committee produced a strategic plan for breastfeeding in the United States that was published in August 2001.

The second operational target of the Innocenti Declaration required the establishment of an agency and a process for ensuring that the Ten Steps to Successful Breastfeeding would be practiced in every facility providing maternity services. This occurred in 1997 with the founding of Baby-Friendly USA[33] to implement the UNICEF/WHO Baby-Friendly Hospital Initiative in the United States.

The Baby-Friendly Hospital Initiative is an international effort developed by the World Health Organization (WHO) and UNICEF in 1991 to promote, protect, and support breastfeeding in hospitals and birth centers worldwide. The program is built both nationally and internationally around a list of ten research-supported practices, the Ten Steps to Successful Breastfeeding, that were developed for maternity facilities.[34]

Following a United States feasibility study that was completed in 1994, an objective on-site evaluation tool was developed to investigate policies and procedures as well as the implementation of the Ten Steps to Successful Breastfeeding. The first U.S. assessment of the implementation of the Ten Steps to Successful Breastfeeding was conducted in 1996.

Regarding the third operational target of the Innocenti Declaration, no action has been taken to effect the aims and principles of the International Code of Marketing of Breast-Milk Substitutes. In an effort to protect breastfeeding, the International Code of Marketing of Breast-Milk substitutes was adopted by the World Health Assembly (WHA) in May 1981 as a recommendation for all governments to regulate marketing practices that promote artificial feeding (formula and other breast-milk substitutes) and the use of artificial feeding devices, such as bottles and "rubber" nipples. The Code was mentioned by then Surgeon General Everett Koop in the opening address to the Surgeon General's Workshop on Breastfeeding and Human Lactation in 1984. Koop established two task forces to investigate U.S. activities and to assess the scientific evidence related to infant feeding[23] in response to the WHO adoption by the World Health Assembly. President Clinton signed WHA Resolution 47.5 in 1994.

In 1990 the national workshop Call to Action also addressed the role of manufacturers with recommendation 12: "Develop a US infant feeding code which states the responsibilities of formula and food manufacturing industries regarding their role in promoting breastfeeding and appropriate infant feeding practices.

1. Convene a meeting of representatives from organizations/agencies and formula and food manufacturers to cooperatively develop and endorse the code.
2. Provide recommendations to federal agencies administering food assistance and related nutrition programs such as WIC (food packages), child nutrition programs, and food labeling.[30]

By the end of 2001, no substantive action had been taken to implement the International Code of Marketing of Breast Milk Substitutes in the United States.

In regard to the fourth operational target of the Innocenti Declaration, no imaginative legislation has been enacted that protects the breastfeeding rights of working women, although in early 1998 national legislation to address this issue was drafted for the first time by Representative Carolyn Maloney of New York.

In November 1998 the National Breastfeeding Policy Conference was held in Washington, DC, by the UCLA School of Healthier Children, Families and Communities, Breastfeeding Resource Program, in cooperation with the United States Department of Health and Human Services Maternal Child Health Bureau. This meeting, referred to as the Barcello conference because of the hosting hotel, developed statements on key policy issues including breastfeeding in the health care system, breastfeeding in the world of work, nutrition and breastfeeding, and the marketing of breast milk and breast milk substitutes.[35]

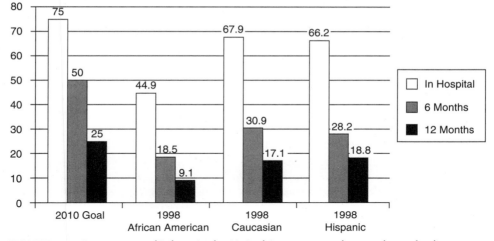

FIGURE 2.3   Percentages of infants in the United States reported as any breastfeeding at hospital discharge, six months, and one year of age in categories African American, Caucasian and Hispanic and Year 2010 objectives.
Data from Ross Mothers' Survey, Ross Products Division, Abbott Laboratories.

U.S. health indicators in many areas including breastfeeding, lag behind those of other industrial countries, and there are disparities in outcomes among groups within the U.S. population.

There is a marked disparity in breastfeeding outcome between women who report themselves as "White," "Black," and "Hispanic" especially at 5-6 months compared to the 2000 goal of 50 percent of women continuing to breastfeed. Only 12.1 percent of "Black" women were continuing to nurse their infants at 5-6 months in 1996, compared to 26 percent of "White" women and 21.1 percent of "Hispanic" women [Figure 2.3]. At every point surveyed, "Black" infants are much less likely to be breastfed, and the gap between the baseline data collected in 1998 and the 2010 goal is greater for "Black" women and infants than for those who are "White." The in-hospital gap is the greatest at 23 percentage points, and a similar percentage (18.5) of "Black" infants receiving breastmilk at 6 months, as "White" and "Hispanic" infants receiving breastmilk at one year (17.1 and 18.8 percent respectively). Clearly, there is a significant disparity in outcome between the surveyed groups. The Health and Human Services *Blueprint for Action on Breastfeeding* mentions this disparity as an important issue to be addressed by breastfeeding promotion projects.[36] The United States Breastfeeding Committee National Agenda also considers disparities a focal activity for achieving U.S. breastfeeding goals.[37]

The United States has developed and become signatory to public policy strategies designed to increase breastfeeding initiation and duration. These policies, including the Innocenti Declaration and statements by professional associations, have repeatedly echoed the desire for breastfeeding to be the normal feeding method for infants and young children in the United States. Unfortunately, policy implementation has lagged behind policy development.

Formula use without medical indication for breastfed babies has increased with more babies receiving formula in the hospital than those who do not. Disparities in outcome mean that identifiable populations are not accessing the irrefutable health benefits of breastfeeding. It is not enough to strategize and plan. The substantive advantages of breastfeeding make the accomplishment of these goals imperative if we are to achieve "health for all" and reclaim breastfeeding in the United States.

References

1. Cunningham, A. S. 1995. Breastfeeding: Adaptive behavior for child health and longevity. In *Breastfeeding: Biocultural perspectives,* ed. P. Stuart-Macadam and K. Dettwyler, New York: Aldine de Gruyter. 234.
2. Ho, M. S. et al. 1990. Diarrheal deaths in American children. *JAMA* 260:3281.
   Schlesselmann, J.J. 1982. *Case-Control Studies.* New York: Oxford University Press.
3. Koletzko, S. et al. 1989. Role of infant feeding practices in development of Crohn's disease in childhood. *BMJ* 298, 1617.
   Koletzko, S. et al. 1990. Effect of infant feeding practices on the development of Crohn's disease in childhood. In *Breastfeeding, Nutrition, Infection and Infant Growth in Developed and Emerging Countries.* eds. S. Atkinson et al. Newfoundland, Canada: Biomedical Publishers and Distributors Limited.
   Rigas, A. et al. 1993. Breastfeeding and maternal smoking in the etiology of Crohn's disease and ulcerative colitis in childhood. *Ann. Epidemiol.* 3:387.
   Greco, L. et al. 1988. Case control study on nutritional risk factors in celiac disease. *J. Ped. Gastro. Nutr.* 7:395.
4. Cunningham, A. S. et al. 1991. Breastfeeding and health in the 1980s: A global epidemiologic review. *J. Peds.* 118:659.
5. Teele, D. et al. 1989. Epidemiology of otitis media during the first seven years of life in children in greater Boston: A prospective, cohort study. *J. Infect. Dis.:* 160:83.
   Duffy, L. et al. 1997. Exclusive breastfeeding protects against bacterial colonization and day care exposure to otitis media. *Peds.* 100:e7.
6. Fallot, M. E. et al. 1980. Breastfeeding reduces incidence of hospital admission for infections in infants. *Peds.* 65:1121.

7. Mayer, E. J. 1988. Reduced risk of IDDM among breastfed children: The Colorado IDDM Registry. *Diabetes* 37:1625.

8. Davis, M. K. 1988. Infant feeding and childhood cancer. *Lancet* August 13:365.
   Shu, X. O. et al. 1995. Infant breastfeeding and the risk of childhood lymphoma and leukemia. *Int. J. Epidemiol.* 24:27.
   Shu, X. O. et al. 1992. Breastfeeding and risk of childhood acute leukemia. *J. Natl.Cancer Inst.* 91:20, 1765.

9. Freudenheim, D. D. et al. 1994. Exposure to breastmilk in infancy and the risk of breast cancer. *Epidem.* 5:324.

10. Zhen, T. et al. 2000. Lactation reduces breast cancer in Shandong Province, China. *Am. J. Epidem.* 152(12):1129.

11. Piscane, A. N. et al. 1994. Breastfeeding and multiple sclerosis. *BMJ* 308:1411.

12. Saarinen, U., and M. Kojosaari. 1995. Breastfeeding as prophylaxis for atopic disease. *Lancet* 346:1065.

13. von Kries, R. et al. 1999. Breastfeeding and obesity: Cross sectional study. *Br. Med. J.* 319:147.

14. Robert, J. L. 1990. Does breastfeeding protect the hypothyroid infant whose condition is diagnosed by newborn screening? *AJDC* 144:319.

15. Rogan, W. J., and B. C. Gladden. 1993. Breastfeeding and cognitive development. *Early Hum. Devel.* 31:181.

16. Lucas, A. et al. 1998. Randomised trial of early diet in preterm babies and later intelligence quotient. *Br. Med. J.* 317(7171):1481.

17. Birch, E. 1993. Breastfeeding and optimal visual development. *J. Ped. Opthmol. Strabismus* 30:33.

18. Temboury, M. C. et al. 1994. Influence of breastfeeding on the infant's intellectual development. *J. Ped. Gastr. Nutr.* 18:31.

19. Kramer, F. M. et al. 1993. Breastfeeding reduced maternal lower body fat. *JADA* 93(4):429.

20. Kalkwarf, H. J. et al. 1996. Intestinal calcium absorption of women during lactation after recovery after weaning. *Am. J. Clin. Nutr.* 63:526.

21. Cumming, R. G., and R. J. Klineberg. 1993. Breastfeeding and other reproductive factors and the risk of hip fractures in elderly women. *Int. J. Epidemiol.* Aug. 22(4):684.

22. Lawson, M. 1998. Recent trends in infant nutrition. *Nutrition* 14:755.

23. Koop, C. E. 1984. Keynote Address. In *Report of the Surgeon General's Workshop on Breastfeeding and Human Lactation.* Rochester, NY, 3.

24. United States Department of Health and Human Services (USDHHS).1980. *Promoting health, preventing disease: Objectives for the nation.* Rockville, MD: Department of Health and Human Services,75.

25. Spisak, S., and S. S. Gross. 1991.*Second follow-up report: The Surgeon General's workshop on breastfeeding and human lactation.* Washington D.C.: National Center for Education in Maternal and Child Health.

26. United States Department of Health and Human Services (USDHHS). Public Health Service. 1990. Healthy People 2000: National Promotion and Disease Prevention Objectives. Washington DC: Author.

27. United States Department of Health and Human Services (USDHHS). Public Health Service. 1995. Healthy People 2000 Midcourse Review and Revisions.

28. United States Department of Health and Human Services (USDHHS). Public Health Service. 2000.

29. United States Department of Health and Human Services (USDHHS). Public Health Service, Health Resources and Services Administration, Maternal Child Health Bureau. 1997. *Child Health USA '96-'97.* Washington DC: Author.

30. Sharbaugh, C. S. 1990. *Call to action: Better nutrition for mothers, children, and families.* Washington DC: National Center for Education in Maternal and Child Health.

31. Ryan, A. S. et al. 1999. *Breastfeeding trends in the United States.* Columbus, OH: Ross Products Division, Abbott Laboratories.

32. United Nations Children's Fund(UNCF), 1990. Innocenti Declaration on the Protection, Promotion and Support of Breastfeeding, Florence, Italy, 1 August. New York: UNICEF.

33. Baby-Friendly USA. [8 Jan Sebastian Way #13, Sandwich, MA 02563, 508-888-8092] Cynthia Turner-Maffei, National Coordinator, and Karin Cadwell, Convener.

34. Kyenkya-Isabrrye, M. 1990. UNICEF launches the Baby-Friendly Hospital Initiative. *Am. J. Maternal Child Nursing* 17:177.

35. Report of the National Breastfeeding Policy Conference(RNBPC). 1998. Presented by UCLA Center for Healthier Children, Families and Communities in cooperation with the United States Department of Health and Human Services, Health Resources and Services Administration, Maternal and Child Health Bureau. Washington DC: Radisson Barcelo Hotel. November 12–13, 1998.

36. Unites States Department of Health and Human Services(USDHHS). 2000. *HHS Blueprint for Action on Breastfeeding.* Washington DC: United States Department of Health and Human Services, Office on Women's Health.

37. United States Breastfeeding Committee (USBC). 2001. *Breastfeeding in the United States:* A national agenda. Rockville, MD: United States Department of Health and Human Services, Health Resources and Services Administration, Maternal and Child Health Bureau.

CHAPTER THREE

USING THE BABY-FRIENDLY HOSPITAL INITIATIVE TO DRIVE POSITIVE CHANGE

Cindy Turner–Maffei, M.A., I.B.C.L.C.

Baby-Friendly Hospital Initiative

The Baby-Friendly Hospital Initiative (BFHI) is an international program that links breastfeeding with current American health care themes of quality improvement, evidence-based practice, and family-centered care. Created in 1991 by the World Health Organization (WHO) and the United Nations Children's Fund (UNICEF), the Baby-Friendly Hospital Initiative recognizes hospitals and birth centers that have fully implemented ten important steps to successful breastfeeding, outlined in *Ten Steps to Successful Breastfeeding,* first published in 1989 by UNICEF and WHO Table 3.1 lists the steps as amended for use in the United States.[1]

The Initiative was inspired by the Innocenti Declaration, the summary statement of the 1990 international policymaker's conference that listed four operational targets to be implemented worldwide, including the practice of the *Ten Steps to Successful Breastfeeding* by all maternity hospitals and centers.[2] (*see* Appendix A.) The Initiative also incorporates another target of the Innocenti Declaration by monitoring compliance of participating hospitals and birth centers with the International Code of Marketing of Breast-milk Substitutes (also known as the "WHO Code") (*see* Appendix B.)[3]

TABLE 3.1   Ten Steps to Successful Breastfeeding* as Amended for the United States

UNICEF and World Health Organization, 1989

Every facility providing maternity services and care for newborn infants should:

1. Have a written breastfeeding policy that is routinely communicated to all health care staff.
2. Train all health care staff in skills necessary to implement this policy.
3. Inform all pregnant women about the benefits and management of breastfeeding.
4. Help all mothers initiate breastfeeding within one hour of birth.
5. Show mothers how to breastfeed and how to maintain lactation even if they should be separated from their infants.
6. Give newborn infants no food or drink other than breastmilk, unless *medically* indicated.
7. Practice rooming-in—allow mothers and infants to remain together—24 hours a day.
8. Encourage breastfeeding on demand.
9. Give no artificial teats or pacifiers.
10. Foster the establishment of breastfeeding support groups and refer mothers to them on discharge from the hospital or clinic.

*As amended for use in the United States
Source: Baby-Friendly USA

As of 2001, there were more than 16,000 fully designated Baby-Friendly hospitals and maternity centers throughout the world. Comparatively, the United States had designated 32 hospitals and birth centers by mid-2001. In addition, as of that time, 50 facilities in the United States participated in the Initiative through the Certificate of Intent Program. More than 3,000 hospitals and birth centers in the United States are eligible for the award.

Baby-Friendly USA

In the United States the Baby-Friendly Hospital Initiative is administered by Baby-Friendly USA, a nonprofit corporation. In 1997 the United States Committee for UNICEF (now the United States Fund for UNICEF) announced its partnership with the Healthy Children 2000 Project, Inc., in the creation of Baby-Friendly USA.[4] Previously the implementation of the Baby-Friendly Hospital Initiative in the United States was the subject of a feasibility study conducted by an Expert Work Group convened by the National Healthy Mothers, Healthy Babies Coalition, with support from the United States Department of Health and Human Services.[5] The Expert Work Group was convened in 1992 and completed its deliberations in 1994. During that time, the United States Committee for UNICEF and consultant Minda Lazarov kept the U.S. Initiative alive by creating a Certificate of Intent Program, through which hospitals and birth centers could register their intent to pursue designation. Wellstart International developed evaluation guidelines, criteria, and assessment tools for the U.S. Initiative and piloted the 1996 assessment of Evergreen Medical Center of Kirkland, Washington, the first U.S. birth facility to receive the Baby-Friendly designation.[6]

The philosophic touchstones of the United States Baby-Friendly Hospital Initiative are objectivity, inclusivity, accessibility, voluntary, and celebratory.

Objectivity: The Initiative is based on objective on-site assessment of compliance with the Ten Steps to Successful Breastfeeding.
Inclusivity: All hospitals with maternity facilities as well as freestanding birth centers may participate in the Initiative.
Accessibility: Information and technical assistance are available to all participating facilities.
Voluntary: Birth facilities seek and implement this program on their own, rather than having change forced on them.
Celebratory: Baby-Friendly USA celebrates the achievements of facilities and gives positive reinforcement to those involved in optimizing breastfeeding practices.

The goals of the Baby-Friendly Hospital Initiative are convergent with findings of several United States maternal health documents and campaigns, described here.

Recommendations of the 1984 Surgeon General's Workshop on Breastfeeding and Human Lactation:[7]

Improve professional education about human lactation and breastfeeding.
Develop public education and promotional efforts.
Strengthen the support for breastfeeding in the health care system.
Develop a broad range of support services in the community.

The United States Department of Agriculture's 1996 Nutrition Action Themes[8]

(5.1) Build multisectoral partnerships with a commitment to build a social culture supportive of breastfeeding.
(5.2) Regularly update nutrition components of established programs.
(5.3) Use state-of-the-art methods and technology.
(5.4) Expand proven interventions to fully reach the target groups.
(5.5) Improve policy action through research.

Call to Action: Better Nutrition for Mothers, Children & Families[9]

(11.1) Promote breastfeeding as the preferred method of infant feeding.

(11.2) Continue efforts to develop more effective strategies to promote breastfeeding through hospitals, MCH, WIC, etc.

(11.3) Explore ways to promote breastfeeding through community efforts.

(11.5) Assure that health care professional who interact with pregnant women. . . communicate breastfeeding as the norm.

(11.8) Provide lactation management training to all health care professionals who interact with pregnant and breastfeeding women to enhance their ability to support breastfeeding, and involve hospitals in networking for the promotion of breastfeeding.

The Healthy People 2010 Goals[10]

(16.19) Increase the proportion of mothers who breastfeed their babies. Target and baseline:

Objective	Increase in Mothers who Breastfeed	1998 Baseline	2010 Target
16-19a	In early postpartum period	64%	75%
16-19b	At 6 months	29	50
16-19c	At 1 year	16	25

Using the Baby-Friendly Hospital Initiative to Effect Change

Data available from Ross Laboratories Mothers' Survey indicates that in 1998 the breastfeeding initiation rate nationwide was 64.3 percent, with a 28.6 percent duration rate at five to six months postpartum.[11] Rates of breastfeeding vary considerably according to region, socio-economic status, and ethnicity. The 1997 WIC Infant Feeding Practices Study reported rates of 56 percent initiation and 25 percent duration at six months postpartum among low- and moderate-income mothers participating in the Federal Special Supplemental Food Program for Women, Infants and Children (WIC).[12] Women of low and moderate income are among those least likely to initiate and continue breastfeeding their babies. Ironically, breastfeeding rates are lowest today among those families who could most benefit from the positive health, nutrition, economic, and empowerment outcomes of breastfeeding.

Factors influencing women's choices regarding breastfeeding are myriad. Preconceptual and prenatal breastfeeding promotion activities need to be carefully tailored to the women's concerns. However, even women who choose, or are persuaded to choose, breastfeeding may be dissuaded by negative events during the peripartum period. One study of a WIC population reported that 68 percent of women interviewed prenatally planned to breastfeed exclusively, yet only 20 percent of these women were actually breastfeeding exclusively upon discharge from the hospital and only 17 percent exclusively breastfed after discharge.[13] Experiences of women during the sensitive period around their time of giving birth have great ramifications upon their subsequent breastfeeding activities.[14]

The potential impact of the hospital environment on breastfeeding is brought into sharp focus by the WIC Infant Feeding Practices Study:

> Mothers experience a variety of circumstances in the hospital that are unsupportive of the establishment of breastfeeding. Something other than breastmilk as the first feeding, delayed timing of first breastfeeding, lack of rooming-in arrangements and hospital gift packages that contain formula, bottle, or a pacifier, are examples of neonatal circumstances that may be unsupportive of the establishment of breastfeeding. Only twenty-nine percent of WIC mothers give their infants breastmilk as the first feeding. Sixty percent of WIC infants receive formula as the first feeding and 10 percent receive either sugar water or plain water . . . . Seventy-two percent of WIC infants sleep away from their mothers at least for one night during their hospital stay. Ninety-three percent of WIC mothers receive a gift package from the hospital. The gift packages of almost all WIC mothers contain items that are detrimental to the establishment of breastfeeding, such as formula, a bottle, or a pacifier. Among the mothers who receive a gift package, 86 percent get some formula in the package . . . . (T)hree quarters of breastfeeding mothers experience one or more nursing problems while they are still in the hospital. However, 33 percent of the mothers who experience nursing problems in the hospital receive no help from the hospital staff.[15]

These results are diametrically opposed to the Healthy People goals. The Healthy People goals include targets to reduce the economic, racial, and ethnic disparities in breastfeeding. WIC participants represent a diversity of low-income families, and breastfeeding rates are lowest in these populations. It is unfortunate that the breastfeeding intentions of these mothers are often negatively influenced by outdated practices. Often the negative effect of practices is not visible to maternity staff, who rarely have contact with mothers after discharge and therefore may have no knowledge of negative outcomes.

Mothers learn how to interact with their babies through the modeling behavior of maternity staff; this is particularly important for mothers' management of breastfeeding. The research of Reiff and Essock-Vital indicates that "Learning through modeling was more effective in shaping mothers' early infant-feeding choices than learning through verbal teaching."[16] Therefore, maternity staff must be aware that potential effects of actions may be greater than that of words.

All of the negative practices identified in the WIC Infant Feeding Practices study excerpted above articulate with the Ten Steps to Successful Breastfeeding. Therefore, the Baby-Friendly Hospital Initiative provides a platform for examining and improving breastfeeding policies, practices, and experiences. The Ten Steps to Successful Breastfeeding are supported by a body of research demonstrating the positive impact of each step.[17,18,19,20] Because this material comes from the World Health Organization and UNICEF, esteemed international sources, it may be regarded with more respect than initiatives originating from lesser-known or more local or politicized sources.

The Journey Toward Baby-Friendly Designation

Hospitals and birth centers often begin the successful journey toward Baby-Friendly designation by establishing a multidisciplinary team. The team may include representation from administration, marketing, quality improvement, women's health services, and medical and nursing staff members. The team then may request an information packet from the Baby-Friendly USA office.[21] Team members may review and complete the Hospital Self-Appraisal Tool included in the packet. A thorough, honest completion of this form should identify both areas in which the facility is already doing well with breastfeeding and areas of weakness. The team may review the tool together in order to provide opportunities to explore the beliefs and opinions of team members, and they may find that their initial meetings were largely focused on educating themselves about current breastfeeding practices and literature.

Once the tool is completed, it is recommended that the team celebrate the breastfeeding strengths of the facility. Next, the team prioritizes and lists the areas of challenge, beginning with those easiest to accomplish or most fundamental and continuing with those most difficult or obscure. The team then begins to establish a plan for the completion of the steps in order as they appear on the list. For example, many facilities find that steps such as rewriting policies, improving staff and patient education, and implementing evidence-based practices are much easier targets to tackle than are other steps such as the establishment of a business relationship with the formula vendors (including the purchase of formula or removing pacifiers from well-baby units). Once stronger policies are established, staff and patients are better educated about breastfeeding, practices such as skin-to-skin contact are routinely implemented, and the breastfeeding rate soars, which may surprise team members and staff. With a much smaller percentage of mothers choosing formula for their babies, the cost of formula purchase is markedly decreased. *Barriers & Solutions to the Global Ten Steps to Successful Breastfeeding* addresses strategies that have been used to overcome this and other barriers to successful implementation of the Ten Steps.[22]

Involvement by physicians and administrations has been crucial to success in many facilities. In writing of Boston Medical Center's journey, Merewood and Philipp state, "We have come to the conclusion that physician leadership, or at the very least physician commitment to the Baby-Friendly venture, was and is critical to success."[23]

Many facilities have found it beneficial to focus on the quality improvement aspects of the Initiative. Breastfeeding from a quality health care perspective helps to clarify health and practice implications, described more fully in Chapter 4. Every facility that receives accreditation through the Joint Commission on Accreditation of Healthcare Organizations (JCAHO) knows the value of voluntary quality improvement processes.

Hospitals have become interested in the role that women play in guiding the health care choices and decisions of family members and, in turn, developed women's health centers and specialties to focus on meeting the needs of women. The Baby-Friendly Hospital Initiative has great potential to provide high-quality, proactive care for women at a vulnerable time of their lives: the birth and nourishment of a new baby. Meeting women's needs well during this crucial time period may forge a lasting positive perception of the health care facility and personnel.

Facilities that wish to pursue Baby-Friendly designation first apply for a Certificate of Intent. Later, following consultation with Baby-Friendly USA staff, participating facilities may request an on-site assessment. This assessment includes interviews with mothers, staff, and administrators, review of documents, and observations of mothers and staff. Findings of the assessment team are forwarded to the External Review Board, consisting of representative experts from across the nation, who consider the assessment findings and make a determination regarding designation of the Baby-Friendly award. Facilities not designated upon first assessment and external review are encouraged to request re-assessment once the identified remaining challenges are overcome.

Evaluation of Implementation of the Ten Steps

Several small-scale studies have examined how well maternity facilities are implementing the Ten Steps.[24,25] In assessing Philadelphia area hospitals, Kovach found that these hospitals were only partially implementing the four steps identified as key: breastfeeding initiation, staff education, supplementation, and rooming-in.[26] Dodgson and colleagues studied Minnesota hospitals and found that adherence was highest for step 4 (39 percent) and lowest for steps 1 (2.4 percent), 9 (4.9 percent) and 10 (0 percent).[27]

A study from researchers at the Centers for Disease Control and the Food and Drug Administration identifies the synergistic effect of the Ten Steps.[28] Using data from the federal Infant Feeding Practices Study, the researchers were able to identify 1,100 women participating in the longitudinal survey who chose to breastfeed their infants. From survey results researchers were able to explore women's experiences with five of the Ten Steps to Successful Breastfeeding. Only 7 percent of mothers interviewed experienced care in line with all five steps measured. In comparison with them, mothers who experienced no steps were eight times more likely to stop breastfeeding early. The risk factors most strongly associated with early weaning were late breastfeeding initiation and supplementation feeding of the infant. The authors state, "These results suggest that the cumulative effect of these practices, rather than each individual practice, is most important in breastfeeding outcome. In addition, the fact that a very small percentage of women (7%) reported experiencing all five of the Baby-Friendly practices measured in this study illustrates the need to increase efforts aimed at implementing these strategies within the hospital environment."[29]

Clark and Deutsch of Kaiser Permanente's Moanalua Medical Center of Honolulu, Hawaii, the second United States Baby-Friendly hospital, shared their hospital's experience of the Baby-Friendly process in a 1997 article.[30] They cited several strategies for their successful organizational change, including the development of an interdisciplinary team, a prioritized work plan, and early implementation of staff education. The cornerstones of their work were education, policy, and teamwork. The next step was identification of indicators of success. Indicators were measured and assessed regularly, and results were used to make continuous improvements. Emphasis was placed on involving all players, sharing the plan, staying focused on the vision, and celebrating all achievements.[31]

Impact of Implementation of the Baby-Friendly Hospital Initiative

Statistics from around the world indicate the positive outcomes associated with successful implementation of the Ten Steps to Successful Breastfeeding. In China, after two years of BFHI implementation, exclusive breastfeeding rates doubled in rural areas and increased from

10 percent to 47 percent in urban areas. In Cuba, exclusive breastfeeding rose from 25 percent in 1990 to 72 percent in 1996.[32]

The PROBIT study, a large randomized trial conducted in the former Soviet Republic of Belarus, has provided insight into the potential child health benefits of implementation of the Ten Steps.[33] Prior to the study, hospitals and polyclinics, the health centers through which all citizens receive their health care, practiced maternity procedures similar to those practiced in Western communities in the 1970s and 1980s. This difference allows for "greater potential contrast between intervention and control study sites. However, Belarus resembles Western developed countries in one very important respect: basic health services and sanitary conditions are very similar."[34] The study protocol randomized hospitals and polyclinics in two groups: in the intervention group, extensive staff training was undertaken to implement the Ten Steps, while in the control group facilities no changes were made to breastfeeding practices or protocols. Information about the infants born during the years of the study was collected in all visits to the polyclinic for pediatric care. Data was collected for more than 17,000 mother/infant pairs. Compared to infants born at the control sites, infants born at the intervention sites were significantly more likely to be breastfed to any degree at twelve months, and exclusively at three months and at six months. Infants born in the intervention sites had a significant reduction in the risk of gastrointestinal tract infections and atopic eczema, but no significant reduction in respiratory tract infection. The authors conclude, "These results provide a solid scientific underpinning for future interventions to promote breastfeeding."

Benefits of Participation in the Baby-Friendly Hospital Initiative

Clark and Deutsch found that the benefits of the Baby-Friendly hospital fell into three categories: improved care and service to members, utilization of resources, and positive public image. "For us, it has never been about the award or recognition. It's about healthy babies who can grow to be healthy children in nurturing families. It's about a philosophy of care—an attitude communicated by caregivers in an environment of love, assistance, and encouragement."[35]

Facilities participating in the Initiative can reap benefits such as team building; quality improvement; health promotion (with resultant cost savings to health care systems and insurers); customer satisfaction; and local, national, and international recognition of achievement. Through their work to implement the Ten Steps to Successful Breastfeeding, hospitals and birth centers strive to meet the needs of each new mother and baby with state-of-the-art care that does not interfere in the development of the breastfeeding relationship, thereby assisting in the growth of stronger, healthier families and communities.

References

1. World Health Organization and United Nations Children's Fund (WHO and UNCF). 1989. *Protecting, Promoting and Supporting Breastfeeding: The Special Role of Maternity Services*. Geneva: WHO.
2. United Nations Children's Fund (UNCF). 1990. *Innocenti Declaration on the Protection, Promotion and Support of Breastfeeding*, Florence, Italy, 1 August, 1990. New York: UNICEF.
3. World Health Organization (WHO). 1981 and subsequent resolutions. *International Code of Marketing of Breast Milk Substitutes*. Geneva: WHO.
4. United States Committee for UNICEF (US Comm. for UNICEF). 1997. *U.S. Infants at Risk of Suffering Lifelong Chronic Illnesses*. New York: Author.
5. Lazarov, M. et al. 1993. The Baby Friendly Hospital Initiative: United States Activities. *J. Hum. Lact.* 9(2):74.
6. In the United States, the terms "Baby-Friendly" and "Baby-Friendly Hospital Initiative" and associated logos are trademarks of the United States Committee for UNICEF.
7. Spisak, S., and S. S. Gross. 1991. *Second Followup Report: The Surgeon General's Workshop on Breastfeeding and Human Lactation*. Washington, DC: National Center for Education in Maternal and Child Health.
8. United States Department of Agriculture (USDA). 1996. *Nutrition Action Themes for the United States: A Report in Response to the International Conference on Nutrition*. (CNPP-2). Washington, DC: Author.
9. Sharbaugh, C. O., ed. 1990. *Call to Action: Better Nutrition for Mother, Children, and Families*. Washington, DC: National Center for Education in Maternal and Child Health.
10. United States Department of Health and Human Services (USDHHS). 2000. *Healthy People 2010-Conference Edition*. Washington, DC: Author, January 2000.
11. Ryan, A. S., and B. Smith. 1998-1999. *Breastfeeding Trends in the United States*. Columbus, OH: Ross Products Division, Abbott Laboratories.
12. Baydar, N. et al. 1997. *Final Report: WIC Infant Feeding Practices Study*. Alexandria, VA: United States Department of Agriculture.
13. Romero-Gwynn, E., and L. Carias. 1989. Breastfeeding intentions and practice among Hispanic mothers in southern California. *Pediatrics* 84(4):626.
14. Jelliffe, D. B., and E. F. P. Jelliffe. 1988. *Programmes to Promote Breastfeeding*. New York: Oxford Press.
15. Baydar, N. et al. 1997. *WIC Infant Feeding Practices Study: Summary of Findings*. Washington, DC: United States Department of Agriculture.

16. Reiff, M. I., and S. M. Essock-Vitale. 1985. Hospital influences on early infant-feeding practices. *Pediatrics* 76(6):872.
17. World Health Organization (WHO). 1998. *Evidence for the Ten Steps to Successful Breastfeeding.* [WHO/CHD 198.9]. Geneva: Author.
18. Powers, N. G. et al. 1994. Hospital policies: Crucial to breastfeeding success. *Seminars in Perinatol.* 18(6):517.
19. Perez-Escamilla, R. et al. 1994. Infant feeding policies in maternity wards and their effect on breastfeeding success: An analytic overview. *Am. J. Pub. Health* 84(1):89.
20. Saadeh, R., and J. Akre. 1996. Ten steps to successful breastfeeding: A summary of the rationale and scientific evidence. *Birth* 23:154.
21. Baby-Friendly USA. [8 Jan Sebastian Way, Unit 22, Sandwich, MA 02563, (508) 888-8092, http://www.babyfriendlyusa.org]. Readers from other countries will want to contact their national authority for the BFHI.
22. United States Committee for UNICEF. 1994. *Barriers and solutions to the global Ten Steps to Successful Breastfeeding.* New York: Author. Distributed by Baby-Friendly USA. [http:// //www.babyfriendlyusa.org].
23. Merewood, A. and B. L. Philipp. 2001. Implementing change: Becoming Baby-Friendly in an inner city hospital. *Birth* 28:36.
24. Karra, M. V. et al. 1993. Hospital infant feeding practices in metropolitan Chicago: An evaluation of five of the Ten Steps to Successful Breastfeeding. *J. Am. Diet. Assoc.* 93(12):1437.
25. Wright, A. et al. 1996. Changing hospital practices to increase the duration of breastfeeding. *Pediatrics* 97(5):669.
26. Kovach, A. C. 1997. Hospital breastfeeding policies in the Philadelphia area: A comparison with the Ten Steps to Successful Breastfeeding. *Birth* 24(1):41.
27. Dodgson, J. E. et al. 1999. Adherence to the Ten Steps of the Baby-Friendly Hospital Initiative in Minnesota hospitals. *Birth* 26(4):239.
28. DiGirolamo, A. M. et al. 2001. Maternity care practices: Implications for breastfeeding. *Birth* 28:94.
29. DiGirolamo, A. M. 2001, 98.
30. Clark, L. L., and M. J. Deutsch. 1997. Becoming Baby-Friendly. *AWHONN Lifelines* 12/97:30.
31. Clark, 1997, 34.
32. UNICEF Programme Division. 1999. *Baby-Friendly Hospital Initiative: Case Studies and Progress Report.* New York: Author.
33. Kramer, M. S. et al. 2001. Promotion of Breastfeeding Intervention Trial (PROBIT): A randomized trial in the Republic of Belarus. *J. Am. Med. Assoc.* 285:413.
34. Kramer, 2001.
35. Clark, 1997, 37.

CHAPTER FOUR

BREASTFEEDING, QUALITY, AND THE HEALTH CARE SYSTEM

Karin Cadwell, Ph.D., R.N., I.B.C.L.C.

How Hospital Routines May Impact Breastfeeding

Breastfeeding is acknowledged to be advantageous for both mother and baby, although as many as 30 percent of mothers who choose breastfeeding prenatally may be unsuccessful at initiating breastfeeding after giving birth.[1] Statistics from the 1995 Census suggest that approximately half of all infants are born to families eligible for participation in the Special Supplemental Food Program for Women, Infants and Children (WIC).[2] The 1997 WIC Infant Feeding Practices Study[3] investigated the hospital experiences of women who were WIC clients. Of them, 46 percent reported sore nipples, 25 percent reported that their breasts were "too full," 8 percent reported "inverted nipples," and 3 percent reported that their baby had choked while feeding. The women also reported problems with their breastmilk: 39 percent reported "not enough milk" and 24 percent milk that "came in late."

Almost three quarters of the mothers studied in the *WIC Infant Feeding Practices Study* who breastfed in the hospital reported that they had experienced some nursing problems. Interestingly, up to one-third of the mothers experiencing specific nursing problems reported that they received no help for those problems. Among the mothers who breastfed the first time they fed their baby, the mother's perception of problems with her milk became a significant predictor of formula use at the time of hospital discharge. However, if the mothers had received help from the hospital staff to address their nursing problems, they were half as likely to be feeding formula at the time of hospital discharge. Community support was also important. Among the mothers who breastfed at the first feeding, those who reported that they had received advice from WIC staff to breastfeed were significantly less likely to be formula feeding at the time of hospital discharge.

According to Gill, "breastfeeding mothers expect the nurses in the hospital to support breastfeeding by giving help, but, for the most part, the mothers reported that the nurses were not supportive."[4]

By 1980, Winikoff and Baer had evaluated nearly one hundred research studies designed to promote breastfeeding success. "A wide variety of recent studies confirms the principle that mothers offered reliable information from health workers are more likely to initiate and continue breastfeeding."[5] Humenick and colleagues found that encouragement from the childbirth educator was significantly related to first-time mothers' sustaining breastfeeding. Perceived encouragement from other health care providers was generally not related to subsequent levels of breastfeeding.[6]

Winikoff and Baer's evaluation of the literature clearly demonstrated the efficacy of changing hospital routines as a means of increasing success at breastfeeding. In general, "Anything that restricts feeding contact during the first 10 days of life is associated with less successful breastfeeding."[7] Common puerperal hospital practices can have profound effects on breastfeeding. By modifying policies, mothers may receive increased support for breastfeeding. According to their review of the primary research literature, routines that promoted breastfeeding included:

Rooming-in: This routine has been shown to increase the number of women still breastfeeding at three to four months and may increase the self-confidence of the mother fostering a healthy relationship between the mother and the newborn.[8]

Demand feeding with no supplementary bottles: Especially when combined with rooming-in, this routine led to a 60.9 percent net increase in the duration of breastfeeding.

> The undesirable effects of complementary feeding include not only the physiological inhibition of milk secretion due to decreased sucking, but also the implicit undermining message to the mother: The staff feels she cannot meet the baby's needs by herself. This message also may be conveyed by other rigid procedures with equally deleterious effects.[9]

Immediate breastfeeding and skin-to-skin contact: Benefits included up to 100 percent increase in duration of breastfeeding, more affectionate maternal behavior, and more weight gained by the babies at six months and one year of age.[10]

The opportunity for immediate contact may not be sufficient, however. Work by Righard and colleague Alade suggest that hospital routines, such as labor and delivery medications and separation of mother and baby for weighing, eye drops, and the like, may affect the quality of the immediate contact experience, especially the infants' ability to "self-attach." The act of mothers merely seeing and holding their infants briefly after birth and then putting the babies to the breast when they are not ready to self-attach may make an insignificant contribution to breastfeeding support.[11] On the other hand, the unseparated, unmedicated mother-baby pair, left uninterrupted to find the optimum time for self-attachment during the first hour or two postpartum, has a higher probability of proceeding to nurse successfully.[12]

Effect of Anesthesia and Analgesia

Righard and colleague Alade found a difference between the self-attaching behavior of babies whose mothers received and those who did not receive the labor medication pethidine (meperidine). The babies who had the most difficulty attaching were those who had both a medicated delivery and a period of separation for weighing, eye drops, and such during the first hour. Nissen suggests that if the mother has had a medicated labor or delivery, two or more hours of unseparated postdelivery contact are needed to facilitate successful breastfeeding.[13]

In a comprehensive review of research about the use of anesthetic agents and their excretion into breast milk, Spigset presented the reported effects on suckling infants and discussed the precautions that should be considered. Spigset concluded that "to date, there is no evidence that any anesthetic agent used on a single-dose basis to the mother causes detrimental effects in the healthy suckling newborns and infants."[14]

An opposing point of view was presented by Sepkoski and colleagues, who stated, "maternal obstetric medication has been consistently associated with detrimental effects on the neonate's behavioral functioning during the first few days of life." They continue, "Babies delivered to medicated mothers are less alert, with poorer muscle tone than babies born to non-medicated mothers, and have more difficulty in habituating to repeated stimuli until the third day after birth."[15]

The association between the drug itself and the condition of the baby may not, however, be one of cause and effect.[16] Sepkoski and colleagues remind us that the factors associated with the use of drugs, such as "longer labor and more difficult delivery, limited childbirth preparation, lower maternal self-esteem and other personality variables," may play a part in the later behavior of the newborn.[17]

In their study, Sepkoski and colleagues accounted for some of these variables to determine whether low to moderate doses of obstetric medication could affect the newborn's behavior over the first month of life. The researchers found that:

> . . . the use of epidural anesthesia—as the main variable differentiating groups in the comparisons and as a predictor variable in the regressions—was related to poorer behavioral outcome and recovery for the infant over the first month of life. The medicated infants showed less alertness and ability to orient over the first month, and in the motor cluster were less mature.[18]

Ransjo-Arvidson and colleagues examined the relationship of the infant's oxytocin stimulating hand movements after birth and found a significant decline in movement with maternal analgesia use.[19]

Maternal Perception

In response to a systems theory point of view that "problems with feeding affect maternal perception of the neonate and adversely affect the breastfeeding experience."[20] Matthews developed an Infant Breastfeeding Assessment Tool (IBFAT). Matthews continues,

> The results of this study support the conclusions of Bentovim[21] and other researchers who strongly support the need for mothers who experience difficulties with breastfeeding in the early postpartum period to receive nursing and medical support to help them overcome feelings of discouragement.
>
> The early initiation period of breastfeeding has been identified as a critical period for breastfeeding success. The mother's perception of the neonate's progress and satisfaction with breastfeeding and her motivation to continue breastfeeding are either positively or negatively reinforced at the time. The neonate's competence at the breast appears to serve as a primary reinforcer.[22]

In an effort to examine maternal and hospital factors that might explain why so many neonates of breastfeeding women are given supplementary formula, Kurinij and Shiono constructed a study in which they looked at 726 women who delivered their first child in one of three metropolitan Washington, DC, hospitals. Their findings suggest that hospital influences, particularly those hospital practices that delay early initiation of breastfeeding, can promote formula use and indirectly shorten breastfeeding duration.[23]

In a meta-analysis of hospital-based infant feeding practices, however, Perez-Escamilla and colleagues were unable to find a clear impact of early mother-infant contact on breastfeeding success. The authors conclude that the results "suggest that early maternal-infant contact might have a beneficial effect on lactation performance. However, to confirm this finding, additional studies with more rigorous methodology are needed."[24]

The association of subtle teaching messages absorbed by mothers from health professionals and hospital routines has been described by Reiff and Essock-Vitale.[25] After discharge, almost all mothers doing any amount of bottle-feeding were using the same brand of formula and ready-to-feed preparation that was introduced during their hospital stay. It was concluded that "the hospital staff and routines exerted a stronger influence on mothers' infant feeding practices by nonverbal teaching (the hospital 'modeling' of infant formula products) than by verbal teaching (counseling, supporting, breastfeeding)."

Bloomquist and colleagues in a prospective study examined the feeding routines of a maternity unit and the subsequent feeding patterns of 521 newborns. They concluded that the administration of supplementary donor milk or formula during the early neonatal period was associated with an increased risk of short-duration breastfeeding, even after adjustment for a number of potential confounding variables, such as maternal education.[26] They noted that "mothers with diabetes or gestational diabetes [where the supplementation was given on 'medical' indications] did not show any shorter duration of breastfeeding. It might be that supplementation of a newborn on strict 'medical' grounds does not disturb the mother-child interaction and maternal confidence as it does when supplements are given because of 'insufficient amounts' of milk or fussiness."[27]

Kurinij and colleagues found that among black women, the addition of formula feeding to breastfeeding (supplementation) was strongly associated with a shortened duration of breastfeeding. The researchers concluded that more advice and support and less reliance on formula is needed during the hospital stay.[28] Romero-Gwynn found the same relationship in a population of Indo-Chinese immigrants in northern California. Only formula samples distributed at hospital discharge had a significant association with formula feeding.[29]

The Effect of Discharge Packs

Is there a direct cause-and-effect relationship between the availability of formula during the hospital stay and discharge package gifts of free formula samples and the discontinuation of breastfeeding? Naylor writes:

> Although definitive evidence indicating that discharge packs deter breastfeeding may not be available, there is a vast amount of information in the literature regarding lactogenesis, breast physiology

and the development of synchrony between infant demand and maternal supply. There is no doubt that interfering with demand reduces supply and in early lactogenesis, the system seems particularly vulnerable. Obviously, carrying home a discharge pack will not affect this system unless it is used, but the mere persistence of this item as a marketing technique certainly suggests that it is utilized. No sound business continues an expensive advertising campaign that is not effective.[30]

In a study in which mothers were randomly assigned to a group that would receive a formula sample pack at discharge or a group that would not, Bergevin found that mothers who received the formula sample were more likely to have introduced solid foods to their babies of two months of age.[31] "These trends became more significant in three vulnerable subgroups: less educated mothers, primiparas, and mothers who had been ill post-partum. Our results suggest that infant formula samples may shorten the duration of breastfeeding and hasten the age at which solids are introduced."[32]

Formula supplementation in the hospital was associated with a shorter breastfeeding period by Samuels and colleagues. They used a California heterogeneous population for their study. Laughlin and colleagues, in North Carolina, also found that supplementing with formula before the two-week office visit led to the termination of breastfeeding by eight weeks.[33] This decision "was frequently made without medical advice. Nearly 64 percent (14 of 22) of the mothers who added formula within the first two weeks did so without contacting the pediatric practice."[34]

A study of Canadian mothers by Gray-Donald and colleagues sought to avoid "methodological pitfalls" by designing a controlled clinical trial of restricted supplementation. They did not find higher breastfeeding rates at four or nine weeks in the babies from the restricted nurseries.[35] They did find, however, that infants from both groups who were still breastfeeding at four to nine weeks were far less likely to have received formula in the hospital. The researchers wonder if formula supplementation in the hospital is a marker, rather than a cause, of breastfeeding difficulty.

Not every study has found a relationship between formula samples given at discharge from the hospital and successful breastfeeding. Feinstein and colleagues studied 166 nursing mothers for four months postpartum. They found that 83 percent breastfed for one month, 73 percent for 10 weeks and 58 percent for four months or longer. "Breastfeeding duration was not affected by formula samples given at discharge from the hospital. Factors correlating significantly with improved breastfeeding rates include maternal age, maternal education, non-smoking, previous breastfeeding, planned pregnancy, initiation of breastfeeding in the first 16 hours and minimization of formula supplementing." More than one bottle of formula per day, measured at 1 month post-partum was associated with shorter breastfeeding duration. This latter effect was minimized by frequent nursing (seven or more times per day) despite formula supplementation.[36]

In a study of the distribution of formula company materials through obstetric practices, Howard and colleagues found that prenatal exposure to formula promotion materials significantly increased breastfeeding cessation in the first two weeks after birth.[37]

The World Health Organization has prepared the following statement on breastfeeding and the use of water and teas:

> Supplementation in the form of water and teas in early infancy is a common practice and one that is associated with significantly increased risks of diarrhea, morbidity and mortality. On both theoretical and empirical grounds it is concluded that these supplementary fluids are not needed to maintain water balance in healthy infants younger than 6 months who are exclusively breastfed.[38]

Quality Improvement for Breastfeeding

The Baby-Friendly Hospital Initiative is one way to examine hospital policies and procedures that affect breastfeeding, and hospitals are encouraged to engage in it. The Baby-Friendly Hospital Initiative integrates well with hospitals' Quality Improvement processes (QI). The QI process is required in all hospitals that are accredited by the Joint Commission on Accreditation of Healthcare Organizations (JCAHO) and, therefore, is an advantageous way to make change within a structure that already exists in U.S. hospitals.

During the 1980s, the Deming Management Method[39] evolved into quality improvement programs for industry with several names, such as Continuous Quality Management (CQM) and Total Quality Improvement (TQI). Hospitals that engage in the Quality Improvement process find that patient satisfaction increases as quality increases. Hospitals have found that it is possible to engineer dramatic improvements in quality of care through systematic intervention.[40]

A fundamental difference between QI and other change models is the belief that data drives improvement. Without measurement, strategies become activity-driven rather than result-driven.[41] Meaningful, ongoing measurement provides the hard evidence that is needed to make unbiased change. In a QI environment, individual units or cross-disciplinary teams of hospital staff members and community representatives are able to identify problems and use QI tools and practices to improve the delivery of care as related to breastfeeding.

Because the underpinning of QI is total dedication to the customer, the first question the breastfeeding QI team must ask itself is, "Who is our customer?" As Widström and Righard and their colleagues have so dramatically demonstrated in videotapes, the *baby* is the customer,[42] and as Widstrom states, "breastfeeding is the baby's choice." Babies want to nurse after they are born, but hospital practices may interfere with the process.[43] The principles of QI dictate that "all activities of all functions are designed and carried out so that all requirements of all the ultimate customers are met and expectations exceeded."[44] This point of view, applied to the baby who ardently desires to be breastfed, dictates that staff practices and the organization of care are designed to strive toward the ultimate outcome of an effectively nursing baby.[45]

When selecting projects to address in quality improvement studies, components for selection should include those projects that have a high impact on quality and cost, practice patterns that can be changed, and projects that have measurable outcomes. A basic component of QI is the use of various tools to examine and point to the root causes of problems, to state these problems clearly and diagrammatically, and to develop and implement strategies to decrease and ultimately eliminate the problem. This paradigm expects excellence. It is not that *some* babies are discharged having latched on and are nursing well. Obviously, the first limitation is that it may not be the mother's choice. In this paradigm, the hospital staff eventually extends itself to help mothers think about breastfeeding in a positive way, during the prenatal period.

Breastfeeding practices and policies in the hospital are ideally suited to QI targeting strategies: national health goals have been established which expect to improve rates of breastfeeding initiation and duration; fewer women leave the hospital breastfeeding than intended to at admission; and JCAHO supports the use of QI tools to examine and change patient care practices. Quality tools are ideal for examining practices and developing breastfeeding protocols that support successful breastfeeding.

Connecting with the Community

In 1995 and 1996 the author conducted an inquiry into the practices of public health providers who promoted breastfeeding. The research methodology was qualitative analysis of semistructured interviews. Subjects were chosen through purposeful sampling of participants in continuing education programs for health professionals on the subject of breastfeeding in the contiguous 48 states and Hawaii. Volunteers were solicited who were doing a "much better than average job at helping women breastfeed." Twenty-three nurses and nutritionists identified themselves and were later interviewed by telephone. The purposeful sampling of a relatively small sample with in-depth interviews is in keeping with qualitative research designs.

Analysis of the interview transcripts explored how breastfeeding was being promoted and supported on a community level by health care providers who thought that they were doing a "better than average job" at breastfeeding teaching, counseling, or management. Many of the respondents said that they also had been recognized by their peers for their successful breastfeeding support and promotion. Several had been asked to mentor worksite colleagues or develop programs to promote and support breastfeeding. When answering the question, "What kind of interventions do you do that support women who want to breastfeed?" every respondent named multiple interventions, especially the following four strategies:

1. Develop a "buddy system" of peer counselors who call mothers before and after their deliveries. The buddy makes the initial and follow-up calls to the mothers.
2. Have a lactation specialist available as back up for problems discovered during these routine calls.
3. Work to encourage hospitals and parents to bring their babies to breast as soon as possible after delivery and make sure the mothers have competent community support postpartum.
4. Schedule an office visit to assess breastfeeding, preferably before day five.

Other strategies included contact prenatally in clinics with breastfeeding promotion as part of every prenatal contact, visits to the mothers in hospital by community health workers, home visits (including some made by a lactation specialist), nursing mother support groups, and breastfeeding mailers sent to mothers between office contacts. Similarities among respondents included a primary focus on the immediate postpartum period for interventions, rather than a reliance on prenatal teaching. The first posthospital discharge follow-up was always in the first week and often scheduled at hospital discharge. Another commonality was the programmatic use of multiple strategies in order to not exclude any mothers. For example, the program might offer the mother a peer counselor support system, as well as lactation specialists' consultations, nursing mothers' support groups, and home and office visits. Contacts were initiated or planned by the provider, although there were opportunities for families to seek help when necessary. The greatest challenge for these health professionals in order to continue to promote and support breastfeeding seemed to be other health professionals who are not knowledgeable and/or supportive of breastfeeding.

Another significant barrier was hospital policies and procedures that did not foster breastfeeding.[46]

Education in Breastfeeding and Human Lactation

The providers of breastfeeding services vary widely—by discipline, by educational background, and by level of expertise in lactation issues. Those who are trained in a related health care discipline may have had no special education in the field of lactation. A number of lactation helpers have no formal health care training or have been exposed to only brief lactation courses. These diverse backgrounds and occupations among lactation service providers reflects a wealth of insight and commitment. However, it does not assure a common body of knowledge or a consistent high level of service delivery.

Research studies investigating the knowledge and attitudes of health professionals regarding breastfeeding have been published. Attitudes, practices, and recommendations by obstetricians about infant feeding were studied in one New York county. The physicians who were surveyed reported that their training in infant feeding was inadequate.[47] Pediatricians in training were found to have "extremely limited knowledge of breastfeeding management" in a California study.[48] A national random survey of pediatric residents and pediatricians who were board-certified within the previous three to five years indicated that residency training "does not adequately prepare pediatricians for their role in breast-feeding promotion."[49]

An earlier study[50] found that despite the recommendations of the Academy of Pediatrics, almost one-half of the pediatricians surveyed did not routinely recommend breastfeeding. Family practice residents and practicing physicians were surveyed to determine whether they had received adequate training and education about breastfeeding to promote and manage breastfeeding among their patients. The researchers found that many respondents were not only unaware of the many advantages of breastfeeding, but scored low on clinical management knowledge.[51] A questionnaire was distributed to family practice residents in Georgia and North Carolina. Sixty-seven percent of residents stated that their training in breastfeeding counseling was inadequate.[52]

Barnett and colleagues found that "although most health professionals had positive beliefs about breastfeeding, differences by profession, work environment, and personal breastfeeding experience indicate the need for comprehensive training in lactation management."[53] Freed and colleagues investigated the adequacy of breastfeeding knowledge of residents and practicing physicians in pediatrics, obstetrics/

gynecology, and family medicine and found that "physicians were ill prepared to counsel breast-feeding mothers." They concluded, "deliberate efforts must be made to incorporate clinically based breast-feeding training into residency programs and continuing education workshops."[54]

Bagwell and colleagues studied the breastfeeding knowledge and attitudes of dietitians, nurses, and physicians in Alabama.[55] More so than nurses, they found that dietitians expressed a stronger interest in breastfeeding and exhibited greater knowledge of questions asked. The attitude and knowledge scores of physicians were not statistically different from those of dietitians and nurses. In a study of dietitians, physicians, and nurses in Utah hospitals, Helm and colleagues found that dietitians were the least likely to provide breastfeeding information and assistance.[56] The authors conclude, "standard nursing and dietetics training programs have failed to include sufficient education and training to give either of these professionals the proper skills to manage lactation. Nurses, as well as dietitians, must seek out additional education on their own."[57]

Lewinski examined the knowledge base of a sample of obstetrical nurses at three different maternity hospitals.[58] Nurses in the study populations completed a survey of 16 questions testing their knowledge regarding breastfeeding. Only 7 of the 16 questions were answered correctly by more than 50 percent of the respondents. The authors concluded "staff nurses working in OB units continue to teach mothers outdated information related to breastfeeding."[59]

A common base of knowledge and skills is desirable both to achieve the breastfeeding objectives and—equally important—to support the ongoing development, evaluation, and modification of breastfeeding policies through evidence-based practice and data-driven planning. The challenge is to provide members of this diverse provider group with opportunities for training, education, and credentialing that will address breastfeeding issues while promoting personal career development objectives. Naylor and colleagues have suggested three levels of objectives for lactation management education in medicine.[60] These are outlined in Figure 4.1.

Education specific to the field of breastfeeding and human lactation for clinicians and health care administrators and policy makers has been considered by WHO and UNICEF and described and implemented worldwide.[61] Recently, the WHO/UNICEF forty-hour breastfeeding counseling course was evaluated in São Paolo, Brazil. The research indicated that health workers who were randomly selected to participate in the training increased their knowledge and skills related to breastfeeding. The knowledge was assessed three months later, with scores remaining high.[62]

LEVEL I: Awareness

Target Group: e.g. medical students (preservice education)

Example Objective: *Discuss, in general terms, findings from the basic and social sciences of lactation.*
Describe the general benefits of breastfeeding for the infant.

LEVEL II: Generalist

Target Group: e.g. pediatricians, obstetrician-gynecologists, family medicine residents

Example Objective: *Apply the findings from the basic and social sciences to breastfeeding and lactation issues.*
Describe the unique properties of human milk for human infants.
Describe the advantages of preterm milk for the preterm infant.

LEVEL III: Specialist

Target Group: e.g. advanced/independent study, fellowships

Example Objective: *Critique the findings from the basic and social sciences and evaluate their applicability to clinical management issues.*
Discuss in detail the components of human milk and their functions.
Describe in detail the suitability of preterm human milk for the preterm infant.

FIGURE 4.1   Example of Breast Feeding Objectives by Level and Target Group.
Adapted from Naylor, A. J. et al. 1994. Lactation management education for physicians.
Seminars Perinatol 18: 6, 525.

References and Notes

1. Winikoff, B. et al. 1987. Overcoming obstacles to breast-feeding in a large municipal hospital: Applications of lessons learned. *Pediatrics* 80: 423.
2. Owen, A. L., and G. M. Owen. 1997. Twenty years of WIC: A review of some effects of the program. *J. Am. Diet. Assoc.* 97:777.
3. Baydar, N. et al. 1997. *Final Report: WIC Infant Feeding Practices Study.* Alexandria, VA: United States Department of Agriculture.
4. Gill, S. L. 2001. The little things: perceptions of breastfeeding support. *JOGNN* 30(4) 401.
5. Winikoff, B., and E. Baer. 1980. The obstetrician's opportunity: Translating "breast is best" from theory to practice. *Am. J. Ob. Gyn.* 138(1), 110.
6. Humenick, S. S. et al. 1997. Postnatal factors encouraging sustained breastfeeding among primiparas and multiparas. *The Journal of Perinatal Education* 6(3): 33.

7. Kennell, J. H., and M. H. Klaus. 1977. The mother-newborn relationship: Limits of adaptability, *J. Pediatr.* 91:1.

8. Jackson, E. B. et al. 1956. Statistical report on incidence and duration of breastfeeding in relation to personal social and hospital maternity factors. *Pediatrics.* 17:700.

   Lind, J., and J. Jaderling. 1964. The influence of "rooming-in" on breastfeeding, *Acta. Paediatr. (Uppsala) (Suppl.)* 159: 1.

   Bjerre, J., and H. Ekelund. 1964. Breastfeeding and postpartum care. *Acta. Paediatr. (Uppsala) (Suppl.)* 159: 1.

   McBryde, A. 1951. Compulsory rooming-in on the ward and private new born service at Duke Hospital. *JAMA* 145: 625.

   Sousa, P. L. R. et al. 1974. Attachment and Lactation. Presented at the Fifteenth International Congress of Pediatrics, Buenos Aires.

   Clavano, N. 1978. As cited in Winikoff, B. et al. 1988. *Feeding Infants in Four Societies.* New York: Greenwood Press.

9. Klaus, M. H., and J. H. Kennell. 1976. *Maternal-infant bonding.* St. Louis: The C. V. Mosby Company.

10. Lozoff, B. et al. 1977. The mother-newborn relationship: Limits of adaptability. *J. Pediatr.* 91:1. [A later study not included in the Winikoff and Baer review is: Romero-Gwynn, E., and B. Carias. 1989. Breastfeeding Intentions and Practice Among Hispanic Mothers in Southern California. *Peds.* 84(4):626. This study indicated increased breastfeeding success for Hispanic mothers who nursed in the first ten hours.]

11. Righard, L. et al. 1990. Effects of delivery room routines on success of first breastfeeding. *Lancet* 336:1105.

12. Righard, L. et al. 1992. Sucking techniques and its effect on success of breastfeeding. *Birth* 19:4.

13. Nissen, E. et al. 1995. Effects of maternal pethidine on infants' developing breastfeeding behaviors. *Acta. Paediatr.* 84:140.

14. Spigset, O. 1994. Anaesthetic agents and excretion in breast milk. *Acta. Anaesthesiologia Scandinavica.* 38:94.

15. Sepkoski, C. et al. 1992. The effects of the maternal epidural anesthesia on neonatal behavior during the first month. *Dev. Med. and Child Neuro.* 34:1072.

16. Kurinij, N., and P. Shiono. Early supplementation of breastfeeding. *Pediatrics* 88(4):745.

17. "The longer a mother waited to initiate breastfeeding the more likely she was to use formula." Sepkoski, C. et al. 1992. 1072.

18. Ibid., 1077.

19. Ransjo-Arvidson, A. et al. 2001. Maternal analgesia during labor disturbs newborn behavior: Effects on breastfeeding. *Birth* 28: 1.

20. Matthews, M. K. 1991. Mothers' satisfaction with the neonates' breastfeeding behaviors. *JOGNN* 20(1): 49.

    Matthews, M. K. 1988. Developing an instrument to assess infant breastfeeding behavior in the early neonatal period. *Midwifery* 4: 154.

21. Bentovim, A. 1976. Shame and other anxieties associated with breast-feeding: A systems theory and psychodynamic approach. In *Breastfeeding and the Mother.* Amsterdam: Elsevier Press, Ciba Foundation Symposium.

22. Matthews, M. K. 1991.

23. Kurinij N., and P. Shiono. 1991.

24. Perez-Escamilla, R. et al. 1994. Infant feeding policies in maternity wards and their effect on breastfeeding success: An analytical overview. *American Journal P. H.* 84:1, 89.

25. Reiff, M., and S. Essock-Vitale. 1985. Hospital influences on early infant-feeding practices. *Peds* 76:872.

26. Blomquist, H. K. et al. 1994. Supplementary feeding in the maternity ward shortens the duration of breastfeeding. *Acta. Pediatr.* 83: 1125.

27. Winikoff and Baer. 1980. 113.

28. Kurinij, N. et al. 1988.

29. Naylor, A. 1982. Promoting successful breast feeding (letter). *Peds.* 70: 5, 825.

30. Naylor, A. 1982.

31. Bergevin, Y. et al. 1983. Do formula samples shorten the duration of breast feeding? *The Lancet.* May 21: 1148.

32. Samuels, S. et al. 1985. Incidence and duration of breastfeeding in a health maintenance organization population. *Am. J. Clin. Nutr.* 44: 504.

33. Loughlin, H. et al. 1985. Early termination of breastfeeding: Identifying those at risk. *Peds.* 75: 32, 508.

34. Gray-Donald, K. et al. 1985. Effect of formula supplementation in the hospital on the duration of breastfeeding: A controlled clinical trail. *Peds.* 75: 3, 514.

35. The babies in this study were fed on a 4-hour schedule. They were awakened at 2 a.m. for feedings. Traditional supplementation consisted of a routine formula feeding for all babies at 2 a.m. unless the mother requested otherwise. At other four-hour feeding times, infants who had difficulty sucking or seemed hungry after a breastfeeding, as well as those whose mothers had a fever or other postpartum difficulty, also received formula supplementation at the discretion of the nursing staff.

36. Feinstein, J. et al. 1986. Factors related to early termination of breastfeeding in an urban population. *Peds.* 78: 2, 210.

37. Howard, C. et al. 2000. Office prenatal formula advertising and its effect on breastfeeding patterns. *Obs. and Gyns.* 95: 2, 296.

38. WHO. 1992. *Facts about Infant Feeding: Breastfeeding and the Use of Water and Teas.* WHO: Geneva, 4.

39. Walton, M. 1991. *The Deming Management Method.* New York: Putnam.

40. Lebov, W. et al. 1992. *Service Quality Improvement: The Customer Satisfaction Strategy for Health Care.* Chicago: American Hospital Publishing. 9.

41. Schaffer, R. et al. 1992. Successful change programs begin with results. *Harvard Bus. Rev.* 70, 80.

42. *Breastfeeding is baby's choice.* Arlington, VA: BGK Enterprises. 1993. Videotape.
Righard, L. *Delivery self-attachment.* Sunland, CA: Geddes Productions. 1992. Videotape.

43. Winikoff, B. et al. 1980. The obstetrician's opportunity: Translating "breast is best" from theory to practice. *Am. J. Obstet. Gynecol.* 138: 105. Samuels, S. E., et.al. 1986. Incidence and duration of breastfeeding in a health maintenance population. *Am. J. Clin. Nutr.* 42: 504. Cronenwett, L. et. al. 1992. Single daily bottle use in the early weeks postpartum and breastfeeding outcomes. *Peds.* 90: 760.

44. Ciampa, D. 1991. *Total Quality: A User's Guide for Implementation.* Reading, MA: Addison-Wesley, 6.

45. Cadwell, K. 1997. Using the quality improvement process to affect breastfeeding protocols in United States Hospitals. *J. Hum. Lact.* 13: 5.

46. Cadwell, K. 1999. Reaching the goals of "Healthy People 2000" regarding breastfeeding. *Clinics in Perinatology* 26 (2): 527.

47. Howard, C. R. et al. 1997. Attitudes, practices, and recommendations by obstetricians about infant feeding. *Birth* 24: 4, 240.

48. Williams, E. L., and L. D. Hammer. 1995. Breastfeeding attitudes and knowledge of pediatricians-in-training. *Am. J. Prevent. Med.* 11: 26.

49. Freed, G. L. et al. 1995. Pediatrician involvement in breast-feeding promotion: A national study of residents and practitioners. *Peds.* 96: 490.

50. Michelman, D. F. et al. 1990. Pediatricians and breastfeeding promotion: Attitudes, beliefs and practices. *Am. J. Health Promotion* 4: 181.

51. Schwartz, K. 1995. Breastfeeding education among family physicians. *J. Fam. Pract.* 40: 3, 297.

52. Goldstein, A. O., and Freed, G. L. 1993. Breast-feeding counseling practices of family practice residents. *Fam. Med.* 25: 524.

53. Barnett, E. et al. 1995. Beliefs about breastfeeding: A statewide survey of health professionals. *Birth* 22: 1, 15.

54. Freed, G. L. et al. 1995. National assessment of physicians' breast-feeding knowledge, attitudes, training and experience. *JAMA* 273: 472.

55. Bagwell, J. E. et al. 1993. Knowledge and attitudes toward breast-feeding: Differences among dietitians, nurses and physicians working with WIC clients. *J. Am. Diet. Assoc.* 93(7): 801.

56. Helm, A. et al. 1997. Dietitians in breastfeeding management: An untapped resource in the hospital. *J. Hum. Lact.* 13(3): 221.

57. Helm, 224.

58. Lewinski, C. A. 1992. Nurses' knowledge of breastfeeding in a clinical setting. *J. Hum. Lact.* 8(3): 143.

59. Lewinski, 147.

60. Naylor, A. J. et al. 1994. Lactation management education for physicians. *Seminars Perinatol* 18: 6, 525.

61. World Health Organization and Wellstart International. 1996. *Promoting Breast-Feeding in Health Facilities: A Short Course for Administrators and Policy-Makers. WHO/NUTR/96.3.* Geneva: WHO.

62. Rea, M. F., S. I. Vanancio, J. C. Martines, and F. Savage. 1999. Counselling on breastfeeding: Assessing knowledge and skills. Bull WHO, 77 (6).

CHAPTER FIVE

LACTATION MANAGEMENT: A COMMUNITY OF PRACTICE

Kajsa Brimdyr, Ph.D.

Is There a Profession of Lactation Management?

Inherent in a profession is vision for that particular discipline: "socially organized ways of seeing and understanding events that are answerable to the distinctive interests of a particular social group."[1] What is the vision of lactation management care providers? Is there a professional vision?

Lactation workers interact with mothers and babies in a community to increase the incidence and duration of lactation by promoting, protecting, and supporting breastfeeding. Is there a specific way that lactation workers approach this goal? What are the ways of seeing and understanding lactation promotion, protection, and support? How are the different aspects of breastfeeding promotion, protection, and support socially organized by groups or individuals within lactation management? These questions must be closely examined in order to better understand the vision, educational pathways, and work practice in the field of lactation support and service.

The breastfeeding initiation rate in the United States in the early 1970s was less than 25 percent, a decline that began at the turn of the 19th century. Not only were few women breastfeeding, but the skills needed to help women breastfeed were not learned by successive generations of women, skills that had been passed from mother to daughter from time immemorial. La Leche League International was founded to provide mother-to-mother support in the cultural absence of intergenerational support. By the late 1970s La Leche leaders, nursing mother's counselors, and lactation consultants were providing information and support to U.S. mothers.

Beginning in the mid-1980s and continuing through the 1990s, the Women Infants and Children (WIC) Program provided breastfeeding encouragement to its clients through volunteer peer counselors, paid peer counselors, trained nutritionists, dietitians, lactation educators, counselors, and consultants.

As breastfeeding support moved from a mostly volunteer mother-to-mother venue in the 1960s, 1970s, and 1980s to a fee-based service in the late 1980s, questions of accreditation, education, and competence emerged. Who is best able to help a mother breastfeed? Is uncomplicated breastfeeding a medical issue? What role should manufacturers of breastfeeding technologies play in the development of policies and procedures? Should the lactation consultant who helps a woman breastfeed be deemed a "professional"?

Lactation Management as a "Minor Profession"

Glazer[2] has described professions as falling into three groups: the major professions such as medicine and law, the near-major professions such as engineering, and the minor professions such as education.

The major and near-major professions are "disciplined by an unambiguous end—health, success in litigation, profit. . . ." These major professions are grounded in systematic, fundamental knowledge, of which scientific learning is the prototype, and operate in stable institutional contexts. The systematic knowledge base of a profession has four intrinsic properties: It is (1) specialized, (2) firmly bounded, (3) scientific, and (4) standardized. According to Moore, "professionals apply very general principles, *standardized* knowledge, to concrete problems."[3]

Glazer argues that the schools of the minor professions are nonrigorous and dependent on representations of academic disciplines. The minor professions are unable to develop a base of systematic, scientific professional knowledge largely because they practice in unstable institutional contexts and have shifting ambiguous ends.

The profession of lactation management or consulting, like education and midwifery, should be categorized as a minor profession. It integrates and overlaps between existing professions. It does not have a specialized, focused, or required knowledge base. In addition, the limits of the profession are not firmly bound, but are inclusive of a variety of experiences, educations, and backgrounds. It is often considered as much an art as a science. Finally, it is not standardized from hospital to WIC program, nor from pediatrician to pump vendor.

Three Levels of Professional Education

Another definition of a profession is offered by Schein in his book, *Professional Education*. He puts forth three properties of professional knowledge:

1. An underlying discipline or basic science component, upon which the practice rests or from which it is developed.
2. An applied science or "engineering" component from which many of the day-to-day diagnostic procedures and problem solutions are derived.
3. A skills and attitudinal component that concerns the actual performance of services to the client using the underlying basic and applied knowledge.[4]

Edgar Schein studied professional education and described the dominant circular pattern of *science core, applied science elements,* and *practicum.*[5] An order exists to gaining knowledge in professional education, and this has been institutionalized in professional curricula. First is the basic and applied sciences, then the theory and technique to solve concrete problems. These are followed by personal skill development in the real world, the practicum that is expected to bridge the gap between classroom knowledge and real world practice. In a profession of lactation management, it would be expected that members of the profession would learn these levels of education in this order, building successively in a strengthening spiral.

Does lactation management or consulting satisfy these three properties? Do workers obtain professional education through this strengthening spiral? Much research has been done on the physiological processes of milk development, letdown, hormones, milk composition, and the effect of breastmilk on developing infants. Do all lactation workers rest their practice on this scientific foundation? Does the community as a whole take responsibility for the comprehension of the basic scientific component of lactation for all novice and experienced workers?

Further, are the day-to-day diagnostic procedures consistent throughout the profession? Are problem solutions consistently taught to all novices? Do the members of the profession agree on these diagnostic and problem solutions?

It must also be asked, are there specific skills and attitudes taught to novices, employed by experts, and endorsed by the professional community? How are they taught? How are they refined?

TABLE 5.1   Lactation Education According to WHO/UNICEF

Course Title	Goal	Target Group	Length
Promoting Breastfeeding in Health Facilities: A Short Course for Administrators and Policy Makers	To sensitize administrators and directors of health facilities to the importance of breastfeeding and the Baby-Friendly Hospital Initiative	Health facility directors and administrators	10 to 12–hour course
Breastfeeding Management and Promotion: An 18-Hour Course for Maternity Staff	To change maternity care to be breastfeeding-friendly	All staff of a maternity facility	18-hour course +3 hours of clinical practice
Breastfeeding Counseling: A Training Course	To develop clinical and counseling skills in breastfeeding	Key health workers in all parts of the health system	40-hour course +8 hours of clinical practice
Training Guide in Lactation Management	To prepare a cadre who can become trainers or Baby-Friendly Hospital Initiative assessors	Trainers, policy makers, doctors, senior community workers	80-hour course +6 hours of clinical practice (40 hours are the Breastfeeding Counseling course above)

Data from World Health Organization and Wellstart International. 1996. *Promoting breastfeeding in health facilities: A short course for administrators and policy-makers. WHO/NUTR/96.3.* Geneva: WHO.

The profession of lactation management or consulting is not yet at the level of underlying discipline, basic science, or applied science. Instead, it is at the level of creating a common base of knowledge. A common base of knowledge and skill is desirable both to achieve the breastfeeding objectives and, equally important, to support the ongoing development, evaluation, and modification of breastfeeding policies through evidence-based practice and data-driven planning.

The challenge is to provide members of this diverse provider group with opportunities for training, education, and credentialing that will address breastfeeding issues while promoting personal career development objectives. Naylor and colleagues have suggested three levels of objectives for lactation management education for physicians (see Figure 4.1). Education specific to the field of breastfeeding and human lactation has been considered by WHO and UNICEF, as described in Table 5.1.

In the United States, classroom hours could be used as criteria following the WHO/UNICEF example to form aggregates of lactation education, as described in Table 5.2.

TABLE 5.2   Educational Programs in the United States that Correspond to the WHO/UNICEF Courses

WHO/UNICEF Course Title (from Table 5.1)	U.S. Course Title	Focus and Directives
Promoting Breastfeeding in Health Facilities: A Short Course for Administrators and Policy Makers	N/A	Currently there is no specific, consistently offered 10 to 12-hour course for system administrators.
Breastfeeding Management and Promotion: An 18-Hour Course for Maternity Staff	18 Hours of Classroom Instruction	WIC peer counselor preparation programs, other peer counselor training, staff training programs at hospitals working on the Baby-Friendly Hospital Initiative. All maternity staff at hospitals that have received the Baby-Friendly Hospital designation have received 18 hours of training and education.
Breastfeeding Counseling: A Training Course	The Lactation Counselor Certificate Training Program, and others	Several 40-hour courses are available in the United States. These courses have a variety of titles and convey several certification designations.[6]
Training Guide in Lactation Management	Applied Teaching Methods for Lactation Professionals, and others	This is a 40-hour course that when taken in addition to the above 40-hour course provides a foundation for teaching the 18-hour course Breastfeeding Management and Promotion.

United States education programs include a bachelor's degree with a concentration in Lactation Management[7] offered by the Union Institute in partnership with the Healthy Children Project. This undergraduate degree with a core competency in lactation consulting includes the 900 hours of precepted internship along with individualized academic counseling, including distance and face-to-face learning. The program has been designed for adult learners with associate's degrees or some college courses, three-year RNs, and those with a high school diploma. Union Institute's College of Undergraduate Studies offers this program so that it is possible for adults around the world to complete their degree goals in a way that is tailored as closely as possible to their needs.

A master's degree and Ph.D. program with concentrations in lactation management have also been developed by the Healthy Children 2000 Project and are now available.

The Discursive Practices of a Profession

Goodwin's view of a profession focuses on the three insignia of a profession and the methods of shaping them.

> Discursive practices are used by members of a profession to shape events in the domains subject to their professional scrutiny. The shaping process creates the objects of knowledge that become the insignia of a profession's craft: the theories, artifacts, and bodies of expertise that distinguish it from other professions.[8]

Within the domain of lactation management or consulting, the subject, or the focus of the events, is the promotion, protection, and support of breastfeeding. It is the responsibility of support and service providers to appropriately shape the events within this domain. It is the responsibility of these workers to develop and use discursive practices, that is, practices that "go [ ] from premises to conclusions in a series of logical steps."[9] The object of knowledge is the event being seen by the worker, in this case, an event involving a breastfeeding-related situation. These events are examined and understood through the vision created by those who work in the field.

To have a profession of lactation management, the members of the work field must create a clear understanding of the relevant theories. What should every member of the profession hold to be "true, false, unknown?" What are the relevant methodologies, scientific evidence, case studies, surveys, or personal stories? Where can new members find this information? The theories of a profession create a central loadstone for new and experienced members to orient themselves.

What are the artifacts or tools of lactation management? Vygotsky described two types of tools, psychological and technical tools, both of which are significant in shaping a profession's objects of knowledge. A technical tool "alters the process of a natural adaptation by determining the form of labor operations."[10] This is what is most commonly known as a tool of a trade. A professional organization understands its own technical tools. Members of the work field should determine the tools of lactation management, that may include specific books, breast pumps, gadgets, and forms.

What are the psychological tools of lactation management? A psychological tool "by being included in the process of behavior . . . alters the entire flow and structure of mental functions. It does this by determining the structure of a new instrumental act (Vygotsky, 1981c, p. 137)."[11] Must a person complete or comprehend certain courses, experiences, and skills in order to encompass the professional vision of the field? Certain theories fundamentally change the vision of learners, bringing them to a level of understanding expected in the field. How is this true for lactation management?

A profession has a body of expertise that differentiates it from other professions. What is the body of expertise expected in lactation management? Where does a professional learn this expertise? Is it learned from a book, personal experience, specific training, or mentorship? Who is the keeper of this body of expertise, and who maintains and protects it? Too many of these questions are currently unanswered, or are without consensus for lactation management to be a profession with discursive practices.

Lactation Management: A Community of Practice

Lactation management currently is a community of practice, rather than a profession. According to Lave and Wenger, a "community of practice," for example, "of midwifery or tailoring involves much more than the technical, knowledgeable skill involved in delivering babies or producing clothes. A community of practice is a set of relations among persons, activity, and world, over time and in relation with other tangential and overlapping communities of practice."[12] Lactation management encompasses the skills required to help mothers and babies as well as the relationship with other communities of practice, such as health departments, hospitals, medical professions, WIC, and nursing support groups. Each community of practice has its own scope of practice, history, and heritage.

Membership in a community of practice helps to shape the interpretation of situations. "All vision is perspectival and lodged within endogenous communities of practice. An archaeologist and a farmer see quite different phenomena in the same patch of dirt (for example, soil that will support particular kinds of crops versus stains, features, and artifacts that provide evidence for earlier human activity at this spot). An event being seen, a relevant *object of knowledge,* emerges through the interplay between a *domain of scrutiny* (a patch of dirt, etc.) and a set of *discursive practices* (dividing the domain of scrutiny by highlighting a figure against a ground, applying specific coding schemes for the constitution and interpretation of relevant events, etc.) being deployed within a *specific activity* (arguing a legal case, mapping a site, planning crops, etc.)."[13]

What is the perspective of the members within the community of lactation management? This question must be answered by members of the community of practice. A lactation consultant observes a woman's breast differently than a certified bra fitter (for example, watches for signs of milk production or plugged ducts, versus cup size, shape, and surgical history). The specific activity of lactation workers is protecting, promoting, and supporting the mother and baby in the area of breastfeeding.

But what is the usual object of knowledge for lactation workers? Is it the same from country to country or from community to community? Is it the same in a country whose hospitals maintain the standards of the UNICEF/WHO Ten Steps to Successful Breastfeeding? Is it working with mothers and babies on basic areas of breastfeeding, such as latch-on, sucking patterns, positioning, etc., or is it handling problems with failure to thrive, mastitis, or other conditions? Is the usual object of knowledge politics, policy, or advocacy? Goodwin emphasizes that the objects of knowledge become the "insignia of a profession's craft."[14] What is the normal situation for a member of this community of practice?

According to Goodwin, the object of knowledge is clarified through the interplay between the domain of scrutiny and a set of discursive practices. What is the domain of scrutiny for lactation professionals? Is it a mother breastfeeding a baby; a woman's breasts; the baby's mouth or sucking potential; hospital policies; the extended family unit; the role of the community; the national agenda?

Once the domain of scrutiny is clear for lactation workers, a set of discursive, or coherent, practices can be used by members of the community to understand and interpret the event being seen. What are the discursive practices for lactation management? How do lactation workers, as a community and as individuals, logically proceed from premises to conclusions about the domain of scrutiny in order to understand the object of knowledge?

Goodwin offers three ways to illuminate the discursive practices within the context of professional activity: "(1) *coding,* which transforms phenomena observed in a specific setting into the objects of knowledge that animate the discourse of a profession; (2) *highlighting,* which makes specific phenomena in a complex perceptual field salient by marking them in some fashion; and (3) *producing and articulating material representations.*" What are the discursive practices of lactation workers?

"Coding schemes are used to organize disparate events into a common analytic framework . . . Coding schemes are one systematic practice used to transform the world into the categories and events that are relevant to the work of the profession."[15] What do lactation professionals classify and into what groups? The first question relates to the object of knowledge referred to earlier. Groupings stem from the object of knowledge. What are the coding schemes of the profession? Are they the same in the United States as in other settings?

A coding scheme is a procedure that is learned and used by members of the community. Schemes can be taught to new members, and carried (physically or metaphorically) to different event situations. A good example of a coding scheme is the form used by archaeology students to describe the color, consistency, and texture of different types of dirt. The use of this form is taught through experiential classes, in which students learn the coding schemes of a profession, as established by senior members of the community. The senior members then can shape the perceptual distinctions into the work practice of the new students.

Some clear coding schemes in lactation management are accessible for members of the community. Hoover's pictures of mothers and babies with different manifestations of thrush illustrates one example of coding.[16] Members of the community of lactation professionals, however, point to numerous videos and examples of poor latch-on, poor positioning, etc., that permeate the learning material of the field. These offer incorrect examples of coding and learning opportunities to novice members of the community. What are coding schemes that senior members of the community can use to shape the perceptions of new members and, therefore, shape the work practice of the members of the community? Who creates these schemes? How do new members learn them? What is the influence of commercial groups, such as pump and formula companies, on them?

Any specific activity of a profession is situated in a "dense perceptual field" of information. "*Highlighting* structures the perception of others by reshaping a domain of scrutiny so that some phenomena are made salient, while others fade into the background." In this way, methods of highlighting allow members of a profession to bring forward elements relevant to the field, while decreasing the importance of other elements. Highlighting helps to classify phenomena, allowing a member of the community of practice to "link relevant features of a setting to the activity being performed in that setting."[17]

What are the relevant events when working with a mother and baby? What elements should be highlighted and stressed as important, and which ones should not be stressed? Who decides for the workers in lactation management what a worker should highlight when encountering a new object of knowledge (mother and baby) within a specific activity (working towards successful breastfeeding)? Who should decide how to highlight this information? How can these methods of highlighting be communicated throughout the community of practice? How are members presently highlighting relevant events in order to draw conclusions?

The third practice offered by Goodwin in order to understand the discursive practices of a community is *producing and articulating material representations*. What are the graphical representations associated with breastfeeding in a given environment? Are there forms for the professional; notes of interactions with mothers; telephone records; peer counselor journals; hospital records? Do standard guidelines exist for anticipatory guidance, postpartum assessment, or assessment records? Which forms do mothers complete? Is there a breastfeeding log or pamphlets and other handouts? Do members of the community use the material representations to collaborate with others in a way that encourages the cooperative work within the community of practice?

Why is it important to understand the discursive practices of a community? "By applying such practices to phenomena in the domain of scrutiny, participants build and contest *professional vision,* which consists of socially organized ways of seeing and understanding events that are answerable to the distinctive interests of a particular social group."[18] Yet, it is significant that discussions about the three elements of coding, highlighting, and material representations lead to no clear answers or a clear picture of a professional vision of lactation consulting or management.

The Work of Lactation Workers

Hairdressers work in a beauty salon. Physicians work in a medical practice or hospital. Tennis pros work on the courts. Where do lactation consultants work? Who helps the mother and baby breastfeed? Is it the doctor, nurse, lactation specialist, friend, neighbor, family, or local support groups? Who actually helps the mother and baby dyad? Where do women go for lactation counseling? What works and is effective when promoting, protecting, and supporting breastfeeding?

Lactation support can be considered invisible. The feminist research concept of invisible work relates to this work because it strives to "understand the social realities of women as actors whom previous sociological research has rendered invisible."[19] The fact that so many of the questions posed in this chapter have no answers emphasizes the invisible world of lactation workers. Star and Strauss offer domestic workers and nurses as two examples of invisible work.[20] Star explains invisible work in the following way:

> Work may become expected, part of the background, and invisible by virtue of routine (and social status). If one looked, one could literally see the work being done—but the taken for granted status means that it is functionally invisible. Work in this category includes that done by parents, nurses, secretaries, and others who provide on-call support services for others.[21]

Lactation management or consulting represents a situation where we could strive to develop a work practice in order to make the work visible.

The work of helping a mother breastfeed properly is invisible. If the breastfeeding is successful between the mother and infant, it often seems easy, natural, and straightforward, requiring no assistance. What, then, is the visible work surrounding breastfeeding? Wet-nursing was visible work, medical interventions are visible, and gadgets are visible artifacts. The failure to thrive and insufficient milk syndrome represent two reasons why breastfeeding becomes visible. This visibility occurs only when something is considered to be interfering with successful breastfeeding. Once the breastfeeding is "made visible," many prescriptions, gadgets, and "solutions" are available to "fix" the problem.

The skill of helping mothers to breastfeed was lost because of its invisible nature—it is difficult to recognize or value what is not visible. However, the goal of successful breastfeeding is invisible. Therefore, the work of a lactation worker, if successful, also is invisible. If all mothers are successfully breastfeeding, why should a hospital have a lactation specialist on staff? Justifying invisible work is often difficult, which is why the work of lactation support may not be adequately funded. Nonetheless, if the work becomes visible only when something is wrong, increasing visibility by decreasing success is not a solution either.

What is the work of supporting, promoting, and protecting breastfeeding? How is this work accomplished? Other fields have a strong understanding of their own work practice. They understand the ethical issues; tasks and functions of their work; the role of interactions, politics, and the governing boards—what it means to be a member of the profession. In addition, there is a professional vision, and discursive, coherent practices to shape the events within a specific activity. Further, there is accountability for actions and interactions.

In order to see the work of lactation management, and to discover where the work effectively happens—beyond the stereotyped job description—it will be important to get close to the work and to examine the everyday work practice in the context of the work life. Suchman warns that "work has a tendency to disappear at a distance, such that the further removed we are from the work of others, the more simplified, often stereotyped, our view of their work becomes."[22]

Barley warns that "unless we begin to examine what people in modern jobs actually do, we run the risk of generating theories and policies that not only lack verisimilitude but may actually prove to be pernicious. It seems unreasonable to believe that people can plan, manage, organize, or even write about what they don't understand."[23] A solution to this problem requires researchers to learn about how people actually work—not their work according to their managers, or job descriptions, but the actual work practice.

Orr conducted an ethnographic study of copier repair technicians and found that the "stereotypical view is that service is about fixing identical broken machines" and that the corporate attitude was that "the technician needs to understand little more than how to follow the directive documentation furnished by the corporation" in order to perform the service adequately.[24] Orr, after studying the work practice of copy repair technicians, found the work to be much more complex, relying primarily on community narratives and "war stories" to fix the plethora of different problems with copy machines in the field. The research found that the ideas about how the work happened and what people actually did were drastically different from the reality. One way to see the actual work rather than capturing the stereotypical view of a job is to conduct ethnographic research.

What is the stereotypical view of lactation consulting or management? What is the reality? An ethnographic study of the work practice of lactation specialists and care providers could reveal whether working with mothers involves answering the same questions to multiple mothers or different questions for different situations. What do lactation workers actually need to understand in order to give effective help to mothers and babies? What works and what does not work? How do people learn about the practice, the coding, and highlighting? Research is required to answer these questions.

The ethnographic study of work aims to examine "mindful practices and communicative interaction" rather than focusing on the cognition of an individual, hierarchies, or other "psychological" or "sociological" aspects of work.[25] Suchman explains the significance of this type of study: "the way in which people work is not always apparent. Too often, assumptions are made as to how tasks are performed rather than unearthing the underlying work practices."[26] Ethnography has emerged as an increasingly popular method of conducting research for qualitative researchers. "Ethnography . . . has become . . . one of the most favored and prestigious forms of conceiving the style in which scholars do qualitative research."[27]

Raeithel coined the term "ethnographic work research"[28] for this type of investigation, which focuses on the "human agency embedded in the everyday actions and interactions of people doing work in various organizational positions and settings."[29]

Ethnographic work research requires a "rapid, cyclical succession of assumption-driven observations—including conversations and interviews—and detailed analysis of documents and dialogue transcripts." This includes focusing on direct observations and informal interviews. Ethnographic work research also includes descriptions of the site, as well as the ethnographer's interpretations of "the formulations of the work practices adopted and used by participants in the organization and change of their cooperative work practices."[30] Raeithel summarizes ethnographic work research by explaining that:

> The application of ethnographic methods to work research, then, begins by our viewing each work group of the organization as a culturally alien community whose world-model and practices we must reconstruct from the utterances and situated actions of the working persons.[31]

Through their focus on the work, people, and interactions, ethnographic work site studies "provide insight into the social nature of work."[32] "The purpose of an ethnographic approach is not so much to show *that* work is socially organized (which is rather easy) but to show *how* it is socially organized."[33] As Hughes, et al. explains:

> . . . the main virtue of ethnography is its ability to make visible the "real world" sociality of a setting. As a mode of social research [ethnography] is concerned to produce detailed descriptions of the "workaday" activities of social actors within specific contexts. It is a naturalistic method relying upon material drawn from the first-hand experience of a fieldworker in some setting. It seeks to present a portrait of life as seen and understood by those who live and work within the domain concerned. It is this objective which is the rationale behind the method's insistence on the direct involvement of the researcher in the setting under investigation. The intention of ethnography is to see activities as social actions embedded within a socially organised domain and accomplished in and through the day-to-day activities of participants. It is this which provides access to the everyday ways in which participants understand and conduct their working lives.[34]

Although ethnographic workplace studies use the same basic definition of ethnography expanded on above, Suchman and Trigg apply ethnography specifically to work practice:

> Ethnography, the traditional method of social and cultural anthropology, involves the careful study of activities and relations between them in a complex social setting. Such studies require extended participant observation of the internal life of a setting, in order to understand what participants themselves take to be relevant aspects of their activity. Importantly, this may include things that are so familiar to them as to be unremarkable (and therefore missing from their accounts of how they work), although being evident in what they can actually be seen to do.[35]

Ethnographic studies of the actual work practice of lactation consulting or management are necessary to understand how breastfeeding can be promoted, protected, and supported. Studies of the process, rather than a specific group of individuals, can help to determine where and how women obtain help breastfeeding. Specific studies of the work practice of people within the field could help to determine the relevant objects of knowledge, the domain of scrutiny, and thereby the discursive practices. We can begin to understand this work only by understanding what influences mothers and babies in the area of breastfeeding.

References and Notes

1. Goodwin, C. 1996. Professional vision. *American Anthropologist* 3: 606.
2. Glazer, N. 1974. Schools of minor professions. *Minerva* 346.
3. Moore, W. 1974. *The Professions*. New York: Russell Sage Foundation. 56.
4. Schein, E. 1973. *Professional Education*. New York: McGraw-Hill. 43.
5. Ibid., 44.
6. Certified Lactation Counselor: The Healthy Children Project Course. Certified Lactation Educator: Lactation Institute, Healthy Children, UCLA Extension.
   La Leche League Leaders (equivalent of 40 hours): La Leche League International.
   Nursing Mothers' Counselors: Variety of programs nationwide consisting of classroom hours followed by mentoring of clinical practice.
7. A bachelor's degree in Maternal and Child Health: Lactation Counseling is offered through a partnership between The Union Institute and the Healthy Children Project. A bachelor's degree in Human Development with a focus on lactation is offered through Pacific Oaks College.
8. Goodwin, C. 1996.
9. Guralnik, D. B., Ed. 1982. *Webster's New World Dictionary: Second College Edition*. New York: Simon and Schuster. 403.
10. Wertsch, J., and P. Tulviste. 1996. L. S. Vygotsky and Contemporary Developmental Psychology. *An Introduction to Vygotsky*. H. Daniels. London: Routledge. 62.
11. Ibid., 61.
12. Lave, J., and E. Wenger. 1996. *Situated learning: Legitimate peripheral participation*. New York: Cambridge University Press. 98.
13. Goodwin, C. 1996.
14. Ibid.
15. Ibid., 607–608.
16. Hoover, K. 2001. *The Link Between Infants' Oral Thrush and Nipple and Breast Pain in Lactating Women*, 4th ed. Morton, PA: Author.
17. Goodwin, C. 1996. 628.
18. Ibid., 606.
19. Reinharz, S. 1992. *Feminist Methods in Social Research*. New York: Oxford University Press. 46.

20. Star, S. L., and A. Strauss. 1998. Layers of silence, arenas of voice: The ecology of visible and invisible work. *Computer Supported Cooperative Work: The Journal of Collaborative Computing* 00: 1.
21. Star, S. L., and A. Strauss. 1998. 12.
22. Suchman, L. 1995. Making Work Visible. *Communications of the ACM* 38(9): 59.
23. Barley, forward to by J. E. Orr. *Talking about Machines: An Ethnography of a Modern Job.* Ithica: Cornell University Press. xiii.
24. Orr, J. E. 1996. *Talking about Machines: An Ethnography of a Modern Job.* Ithica: Cornell University Press. 104–105.
25. Engestrom, Y., and D. Middleton. 1994. *Cognition and Communication at Work.* New York: Cambridge University Press. 1.
26. Suchman, L. 1995. 56.
27. Marcus, G. 1994. What comes (just) after "post"?: The case of ethnography. *Handbook of Qualitative Research.* Edited by N. Denzin and Y. Lincoln. London: Sage Publications. 563.
28. Raeithel, A. 1996. On the ethnography of cooperative work. *Cognition and Communication at Work.* Edited by Y. Engestrom and D. Middleton. New York: Cambridge University Press. 321.
29. Engestrom, Y., and D. Middleton. 1994. 1.
30. Raeithel, A. 1996. 320.
31. Ibid.
32. Hughes, J. et al. 1992. Faltering from ethnography to design. *Computer Supported Cooperative Work.* New York: ACM. 429.
33. Ibid., 116.
34. Hughes, J. et al. 1994. Moving out from the control room: Ethnography in system design. *Computer Supported Cooperative Work.* New York: ACM. 430.
35. Suchman, L., and R. Trigg. 1991. Understanding practice: Video as a medium for reflection and design. *Design at Work.* Edited by J. Greenbaum and M. Kyng. Hillsdale, NJ: Lawrence Earlbaum Assoc. 75.

CHAPTER SIX

TOWARD EVIDENCE-BASED BREASTFEEDING PRACTICE

Anna Blair, Ph.D., and
Cindy Turner–Maffei, M.A., I.B.C.L.C.

Introduction

Evidence-based practice, an emerging model for objectively examining the validity of common health provider practices, entails careful formulation of the presenting problem, evaluation of existing knowledge and research regarding treatment options, and integration of new information into practice.

Today health care workers are bombarded with messages from a multitude of sources, many of which may be of questionable value when subjected to critical appraisal. In the face of an ever-changing and expanding research base, it is no longer advisable to follow a "cookbook" approach to clinical management, that is, to practice as if every problem has a corresponding solution that is always correct and applicable. Clinicians may be tempted to rely on past practice, remembered training, or textbooks for answers to clinical problems. However, by the time new textbooks reach the shelves, new research is likely to have been published refuting some textbook statements. There is a great value in the development of skills that enable efficient review, critical appraisal, and integration of new information and techniques.

Breastfeeding is not a new art. The knowledge of how to best manage breastfeeding in prior centuries arose largely through lay or folk knowledge. Medical and nursing school curricula have included very little information about breastfeeding until recently and then primarily from a medical or problem-oriented point of view. Breastfeeding specialists are likely to have obtained knowledge through personal experience combined with absorption of knowledge from a cadre of acknowledged breastfeeding experts. Breastfeeding specialists may not have a health care background, having been trained through a peer counseling or a mother-to-mother model. Until very recently, little research was published in the field of human lactation, and no standard educational pathway existed for becoming a breastfeeding specialist. A sense seems apparent among some breastfeeding advocates that breastfeeding (the folklore) must be protected from the health care community (medical authority). This perspective may be understandable in light of the iatrogenic nature of many breastfeeding problems (when an illness or symptom is brought on unintentionally by something a physician says or does). Yet it does not promote an optimal environment for interdisciplinary discussion and exploration of best breastfeeding practices. Similarly, authority-based medical practitioners may discredit the observational experience of lay breastfeeding specialists as personal and anecdotal.

The evidence-based practice paradigm can offer tools to address the tension between folklore and medicine by authority and between observed experience and authority. The recent explosion in the publication of lactation research can be of great assistance to those seeking to develop evidence-based services for their clients, as can the availability of more educational opportunities for those desiring to pursue breastfeeding as a specialty. It is our hope that evidence-based practice may help to level the field among various breastfeeding practitioners, providing a forum for interdisciplinary discussion, increasing knowledge of outcomes associated with common practice, and building consensus regarding best practices in breastfeeding care.

Traditional Paradigm: Medicine by Authority

Medicine has traditionally been practiced in an autocratic context following the approach *medicine by authority,* which "rests on the assumption that the authority in question has comprehensive scientific knowledge. Understandably none can."[1] Early societies believed that gods caused illnesses, and since these higher authorities caused the illness, a higher authority would be needed to treat the illness. In the age of Descartes, physicians came to view the body as machinelike, capable of breaking, and needy of repair. This mechanistic view of the body ultimately led to formal tests of medical practices. Nevertheless, medicine's passion for authoritative answers persisted.

The traditional paradigm of medicine by authority was based on four assumptions.

1. Authority is based on the amount of clinical experience of a health care professional. The foundation for diagnosis is built on one's own experience treating other patients. A clinician with twenty years of experience therefore has more authority than a clinician with two years of experience.
2. The scientific foundation for practice is lodged in pathophysiology. The body is understood as a complex machine; pathophysiology is the basis of the repair manual.
3. Clinical experience and personal or collective judgment equip a practitioner to evaluate new tests or procedures. Published research studies are less important than one's own evaluation in this assumption.
4. Mastery of subject areas (as in classroom experience) and clinical experience (as in residency, mentorships, and internships) are the prerequisites to clinical practice.[2]

When practicing by authority, a practitioner has a number of options to draw upon, such as personal experience, what was learned in school about biology, researching the problem in a textbook, or asking an expert. The inherent value is in aligning with accepted scientific authority and strictly adhering to standards of practice. Practitioners using the paradigm of medicine by authority may have difficulty with integrating new research information.

A New Paradigm: Evidence-Based Practice

Evidence-based practice is based on scientific evidence rather than authority, clinical experience, or solely intuition. Evidence-based practice involves making thoughtful, reasoned decisions that integrate well-examined scientific evidence with clinical experience. In order to practice evidence-based medicine, critical appraisal skills are needed. Access to information is an integral part of making reasonable decisions based on critical appraisal. New information and scientific evidence concerning health becomes available every day, and there is a constant need for updating and synthesizing knowledge.

The three assumptions of evidence-based practice are:

1. Outcome measures that have been evaluated and reproduced in a systematic manner can increase the certainty of diagnosis, treatment, and the validity of diagnostic tests. Only when outcome measures are not available does clinical impression

prevail. Clinical impression is, however, regarded as a potentially misleading clue.

2. Pathophysiology is understood as only one part of the knowledge a clinician needs in order to competently practice. Knowledge of outcome measures, risks, interpersonal skills, spiritual life and community support are also important. In this sense evidence-based practice can be more inclusive than observational practice.
3. Formal rules of evidence (presented later in this chapter) are used to evaluate the literature.[3]

Critical Appraisal

Critical appraisal is a detailed process, including the several steps defined below.

- Precisely define the problem through careful interviewing, history taking, and observation.
- Determine what information is needed in order to resolve the problem.
- Conduct an efficient and thorough literature search.
- Select the "best" studies that are relevant to the problem (those with the best research, not the studies that agree with a preconceived "hunch").
- Extract the clinical message from the research.
- Apply the message to the problem.

What are the "best" research studies to guide clinical practice? What published information can a clinician consider as evidence in the evidence-based paradigm? A clinician must critically appraise the article in relation to its validity and applicability. Critical appraisal "comprises the ability to assess the validity and applicability of clinical, paraclinical, and published evidence and to incorporate the results of this assessment into clinical management."[4]

One comprehensive resource for evidence-based practice is the series of articles written by Greenhalgh on the theme "how to read a paper," published in *British Medical Journal* in 1997. Another good resource is the series of articles "User's Guides to the Medical Literature," written by Guyatt, Sackett, and colleagues, published in the *Journal of the American Medical Association* in the mid- and late 1990s.

Hierarchy of Evidence

Guyatt and colleagues (1995) published a hierarchy, shown in Table 6.1, structuring research from most reliable to least reliable.

TABLE 6.1   The Hierarchy of Evidence

Research Design	Definition[5,6]
1. Systematic Reviews and Meta-analyses	Systematic review is an overview of primary studies using explicit, reproducible methods. Meta-analysis is a mathematical synthesis of results of two or more primary studies.
2. Randomized Controlled Trials	Participants randomly allocated to treatment or control groups. Randomized controlled trials with definitive results are ranked more highly than those with nondefinitive results.
3. Cohort Studies	Two or more groups of people are selected on basis of difference in their exposure to a potentially causal agent and outcome is followed.
4. Case-Controlled Studies	Subjects with a certain condition are paired with controls matched for other factors, data is collected, and outcomes are observed.
5. Cross-Sectional Surveys	A representative sample of subjects are interviewed or studied. Data is collected and analyzed to answer specific questions.
6. Case Reports	Anecdotal reports of specific experiences of individuals studied.

Based on Guyatt, G. H. et al. 1995. User's guides to the medical literature. IX. A method for grading health care recommendations. *JAMA* 274: 1800-04 and Greenhalgh, T. 1997. How to read a paper: getting your bearings (deciding what the paper is about). *BMJ* 315: 243.

It is important for clinicians and breastfeeding specialists to be able to identify the relative level of inherent bias in the research they are reading as well as ask themselves the above questions in interpreting the research, extract the message, and apply it to the case at hand. All study designs have advantages and disadvantages. For example, while randomized controlled trials can allow rigorous examination of a single treatment variable, they are expensive to conduct and therefore more likely to be sponsored by commercial interests or to have small sample size. The evidence hierarchy can provide perspective on the merits of various study designs and findings.

Role of Intuition

The use of intuition in clinical decision making poses a challenge in the evidence-based paradigm. Intuition can be an important guide to questioning and developing hypotheses; however, it must be used with caution. It is important for clinicians managing lactation as well as breastfeeding specialists to examine intuitive thoughts and feelings carefully, as they have the potential to be both elucidating and misleading.

Breastfeeding specialists and other clinicians managing lactation may find it helpful to use intuition in guiding the process of interviewing clients and defining and hypothesizing the problem. However, it is important to stop and reflect on the problem and the process before jumping into treatment regimes. After hypothesizing, clinicians managing lactation and breastfeeding specialists must think critically about the information they have and the information that is missing. Many providers of lactation care have had the experience of jumping intuitively from a single complaint to a fairly obscure diagnosis before realizing that very basic potential causes have been overlooked. In evidence-based practice, input from critical thinking, past experience, and intuition are examined and synthesized in assessing problems and situations.

Many, if not all, clinicians and breastfeeding specialists are prone to developing personal attachments to certain treatments. These attachments can form thought filters that block admission of new or diverse information. The challenge is to hone clinical lactation management skills by integrating critical appraisal into assessment and fostering openness to new information.

Obstacles to Evidence-Based Practice

Grimes describes five obstacles to evidence-based practice: seduction by authority, false idol of technology, let sleeping dogmas lie, pursuit of pedantry, and numerators in search of denominators.[7] Application of these potential obstacles to evidence-based breastfeeding practices could be:

- Absorption of the tenets offered by breastfeeding "authorities" as truth
- Absorption of beliefs espoused by those with vested interest (commercial and control interests)
- Unexamined assumptions that certain techniques and products work ("This is the way we've always done it.")
- Lack of dialogue with other disciplines and interdisciplinary nomenclature skirmishes (e.g., "clutch" vs. "football hold," "letdown" vs. "milk ejection," "formula" vs. "artificial baby milk"; etc.)
- Rejection or distortion of research messages in the interest of protecting current beliefs and practices of the field (protection of the "sacred cows")

Many products and techniques in current usage for lactation care have never been studied to examine their safety and efficacy. Some when studied are not only ineffective, but may have a negative impact on breastfeeding outcome. One example is breast shells and exercises advertised and recommended for decades for use in the treatment of inverted nipples. After a large randomized, controlled trial[8] of these devices, researchers found that sustained improvement occurred only in the nontreated control group. Women who were assigned to use these interventions were the least likely to be successful at breastfeeding, and their nipples were no more likely to evert than women with similar nipples who did nothing to prepare them. The publication of this finding in 1992 seems to have had little impact on practice.

It is strongly recommended that practitioners seek and develop an evidence base for all commonly used interventions. Beliefs such as "It's natural; it can't hurt," "Ancient people did it this way—it must be OK," or "This gadget is being sold for this problem; it will help" must be viewed with the same skeptical eye as thalidomide, diethylstilbestrol (DES), and episiotomy. Well-conducted, unbiased outcome evaluation is the best available tool to determine the safety and efficacy of products and treatments.

A Sample Examination of the State of the Research

This passage examines the state of the research concerning a currently popular treatment for engorgement, the use of cabbage leaves applied topically to the breast.

Engorgement is a painful condition defined as "the swelling and distention of the breasts, usually in the early days of initiation of lactation, caused by vascular dilation as well as the arrival of the early milk."[9]

Controversies abound regarding the appropriate treatment for engorgement. Some breastfeeding specialists view the engorged breast as similar to a sprained ankle, thus adapting the accepted practice of treating sprains (rest, ice, compression, and elevation) to engorgement, by treatment with cold compresses to encourage vasoconstriction. Others adapt knowledge of the need for vasodilation to allow the ductules of the breast to release pooled milk and suggest that warm compresses or soaks are more likely to promote the flow of milk from the breast. At this time, no peer-reviewed, widely circulated, objective research data exists indicating a clear benefit to either warm or cold compresses in the treatment of breast engorgement. The lactating breast is neither a sprained joint, nor merely a vascular organ, but rather a secretory organ relying on changes in the circulatory, lymphatic, and nervous systems as well as cellular integrity to provide stimulation and raw materials for the synthesis and release of a unique fluid, human milk. The appropriate treatment for engorgement deserves comprehensive research.

While there is no consensus on its management, it is known that engorgement can be best prevented by immediate suckling of the infant at the breast after birth and frequent, unrestricted nursing with the infant well latched and attached. "The best management of engorgement is prevention."[10]

Cabbage has been growing in popularity as another treatment for painfully full and engorged breasts as is indicated by discourse on LACTNET, a list server of electronic mail for those working in the field of lactation.[11] Cabbage has been identified as an anti-edema treatment in several herbal texts, through folk knowledge, and in the emerging field of *phytomedicine,* which studies the use of plants for medicinal purposes. Knowledge of treatments believed to work in reducing edema on other parts of the body, such as a sprained ankle, have been "transplanted" for use in the treatment of engorgement.

In 1988, Rosier reported nine case histories "where cabbage leaf compresses . . . afforded relief of engorgement." In two of these case histories, cabbage is reported to have suppressed lactation in women who wished to wean. The remainder of the case histories credit cabbage treatment with reversing delayed initiation of breastfeeding, relieving pain, inducing milk flow, and relieving "giant hypertrophy" of the breast. The seemingly contradictory finding that cabbage use can both induce milk flow and suppress milk supply is not addressed. How is the clinician to make sense of this? The proposed mechanism is "an unknown substance . . . absorbed from the cabbage leaf through mother's skin. The effect is firstly, a substantial reduction in oedema and an improved milk flow. However, prolonged use appears to reduce milk supply."[12] Thus, Rosier presents us with the first published case reports of the use of cabbage leaves to treat breast engorgement, as depicted in Table 6.2. New findings are often presented in this format to spur more

TABLE 6.2   Rosier's Findings: Use of Cool Cabbage Compresses   n = 9

2 cases	Suppression of lactation in weaning mothers
5 cases	Reduction of engorgement and establishment of successful breastfeeding
2 cases	Relief of "giant hypertrophy" of the breasts

Evidence Level 6: Case Reports

Potential Flaws: Anecdotal, no control of confounding factors

Based on Rosier, W. Cool cabbage compresses *Breastfeeding Rev.* 12: 28–31.

objective research. It is important to recall that case reports, while valuable as thought and research provocateurs, are on the lowest level (6) of the evidence hierarchy (Table 6.1).

Following the Rosier case reports, Nikodem and colleagues published the first randomized controlled study of cabbage leaves in 1993. In this research, 120 breastfeeding women were randomly assigned to a treatment group (cabbage leaf application) or control group (routine care) at seventy-two hours postpartum. The authors report that the "experimental group tended to report less breast engorgement, but this *trend was not statistically significant.*"[13] At six weeks duration, women who received cabbage leaf application were more likely to be breastfeeding than the control group.

The authors summarized:

> . . . we cannot rule out the possibility that cabbage leaves had a direct effect on breast engorgement . . . however, we consider that the positive effect was more likely to have been mediated by psychological mechanisms . . . . We postulate that the fact that women in the experimental group were actively involved in a procedure perceived to be beneficial to breastfeeding may have increased their confidence and self-esteem, and initiated a positive cycle of success.[14]

This work would be placed on level 2 of the evidence hierarchy, randomized controlled trials. This study also illustrates some of the difficulty of this type of research: while selection of the treatment group can be random, treatment with a cabbage leaf cannot be blind. Women obviously know that something potentially helpful has been placed on their breasts. Placebo effect may be triggered, as well as the women's sense of confidence, as the researchers eloquently elaborate. Table 6.3 displays women's perception of engorgement, according to Nikodem.

TABLE 6.3   Nikodem: Perception of Engorgement   n = 12

Assessment	Experimental	Control	P value
First	54%	56%	.93
Second	51%	57%	.68
Third	49%	51%	.69
Fourth	54%	59%	.73

Evidence Level 2: Randomized controlled trial

Potential Flaws: Unblinded study, self-reported pain index, researcher-identified placebo effect regarding intervention.

No statistically significant differences (P > .68)

Adapted from Nikodem, V. C. et al. 1993. Do cabbage leaves prevent breast engorgement? A randomized, controlled study. *Birth* 20(2): 61.

TABLE 6.4   Roberts Comparison of Cabbage and Gelpacks on Post Test Pain   n = 34

Treatment Group	Reduction in Pain	P
Cabbage group	30%	.0001
Gelpack group	39%	.0001

Evidence Level: Below 2

Potential Flaws: Treatment is comparative (one therapy for each breast) rather than randomized and controlled; no untreated controls; small sample size

Based on Roberts, K. L. 1995a. A comparison of chilled cabbage leaves and chilled gelpacks in reducing breast engorgement. *J. Hum. Lact.* 11(1): 17.

Roberts and colleagues have conducted additional studies to determine the potential effects of cabbage. The first study compared the effects of chilled cabbage leaves and chilled gelpacks in reducing engorgement. Each woman used cabbage leaves on one breast and gelpacks on the other. Each mother completed pre- and posttest pain scale ratings for the breasts. There was no statistically significant difference *between* posttreatment pain level of either treatment. Both treatments resulted in maternal reports of reduced pain, with a trend toward greater pain reduction in the gelpack breast. The "p" values shown in Table 6.4 indicate that both treatments were associated with statistically significant reduction in reported pain. As Nikodem identified, there are two possible causes for this reduction: the treatments and the psychological benefits of treatment. This study is a comparative trial, rather than a controlled one. There was no untreated control group.

Roberts and colleagues published a second study examining the effect of chilled versus room temperature cabbage leaves administered in the same format as the prior study. No statistically significant difference was found *between* the two treatments. Both treatments resulted in maternal reports of reduced pain. The "p" values shown in Table 6.5 indicate that both treatments were associated with statistically significant reduction in reported pain. As discussed above, it is unclear whether the source of pain relief is a chemical or physiological action of the treatment or the caregiving aspects of administration of treatment.

The authors discuss the implication of the finding of no difference between chilled and room temperature treatments on the hypothesis of the unknown substance thought to be reducing swelling and increasing milk flow. "It was expected that if there were no active substances in the cabbage leaves, chilled leaves would give greater relief than those at room temperature. However, if there were an active substance

TABLE 6.5   Roberts Comparison of Chilled and Room Temperature Cabbage Leaves n = 28

Treatment	Pain Reduction	P value
Room Temperature Cabbage	37%	.0001
Chilled Cabbage	38%	.0001

Evidence Level: Below 2

Potential Flaws: Each subject's treatment is comparative (one therapy for each breast), rather than randomized and controlled; no untreated control group; small sample size

Based on Roberts, K. L. et al. 1995b. A comparison of chilled and room temperature cabbage leaves in treating breast engorgement. *J. Hum. Lact.* 11(3): 191.

TABLE 6.6   Roberts Comparison of Cabbage Leaf Extract with Placebo   n = 39

No statistically significant difference between experimental and control group in any of seven indicators, except that both groups perceived creams to have some efficacy.

Evidence Level: 2

Potential Flaws: Small sample size

Based on Roberts, K. L. et al. 1998. Effects of cabbage leaf extract on breast engorgement. *J. Hum. Lact.* 14: 231.

in the cabbage leaves, the room temperature cabbage leaves would show a greater effect because of increased chemical absorption."[15]

Attempting to address the barrier to blindness of mothers and researchers and the placebo effect, Roberts and colleagues conducted a third study assigning women to use either a cabbage extract contained in cream base or the cream base alone (Table 6.6). Breast engorgement was measured by physical observation, measurement using a special device, and the use of two scales eliciting the mother's experience of engorgement. No statistically significant differences were found between the experimental and control groups. Mothers from both groups reported that the creams were helpful; however, the "magnitude of this perceived relief was low and in the range of the placebo effect."[16] After feeding the baby, mothers reported the greatest degree of pain relief. "The implication of the results of this study for practice is that when mothers become engorged, the first priority should be to encourage them to breastfeed their baby frequently if possible rather than to use a remedy whose scientific basis has not yet been established."[17]

The literature presented above shows there is not a single study of high-level evidence that shows statistically significant benefits of topical cabbage applications on engorgement when compared to other treatments and controls. The highest level evidence reviewed here shows no statistically significant improvement of engorgement related to the use of cabbage.

Other studies presented could be criticized for small sample size and lack of untreated controls. As mentioned, the physical appearance and smell of cabbage would make double-blind study protocol difficult. The last study reviewed attempts to remove this bias and shows no statistically significant difference between use of cream containing cabbage extract and a placebo. The study cited in the Cochrane evaluation of the effect of cabbage on engorgement concludes that both cabbage extract and placebo cream were equally effective.[18]

Currently, no research exists to back up Rosier's proposed rationale for efficacy; no anti-edema cabbage chemical has yet been identified. Thus, Roberts summarizes, "Cabbage leaves will undoubtedly continue to be used as a treatment for breast engorgement as they are well received by some clients and do not appear to do any harm. Nevertheless, until a scientific foundation for their action is established, their use will remain questionable."[19]

One could raise the question, "What harm could it do to encourage a woman to use cabbage? It may not do any good, but it won't hurt." From an evidence-based standpoint, it is highly questionable to make claims for any benefits of techniques and treatments that have not been proven. The outcomes of treatments, their safety, and efficacy cannot be determined reliably on an anecdotal basis alone.

Clinicians providing lactation management care and breastfeeding specialists may lose credibility with clients and research-based colleagues for espousing unsupported recommendations. Clinging to anecdotal evidence in the face of little scientific evidence is not the optimal stand for an evidence-based health care worker.

One must think about the possible side effects of the postulated, but as yet undiscovered, antidiuretic agents. If these elusive agents are chemically capable of transdermal passage, the probability of their presence in a mother's milk is high. Another important question is, What effect do these agents have on the infant who consumes them?

Another concern about the use of cabbage is that raw cabbage is known to be a potential carrier for listeria.[20] Listeriosis is a serious form of food poisoning. Certainly clinicians would not wish to expose infants to a potential vector of listeria through use of cabbage on the breast.

Finally, as the last Roberts study illustrates, the treatment often overlooked in the search for the gadget or substance that could fix a breastfeeding problem is generally the best remedy of all: a well-latched, suckling baby.

Conflicts often arise over differing opinions in breastfeeding management. Arguments over the "correct way" to practice can lead to stress and affect patient care. In the field of human lactation, many of these arguments are over such issues as alternative feeding methods, which breast pump is the best, whether the bottom lip should be tickled as the baby is starting to latch on, or even if it is worth it to breastfeed at all. These types of arguments between health care providers could negatively affect mothers and babies. Analyzing the existing evidence regarding the options can provide a level field for discussion and collaborative decision making.

References

1. Grimes, D. A. 1995. Introducing evidence-based medicine into a department of obstetrics and gynecology. *Obstet. Gyn.* 86(3): 451.
2. Ibid., 452.
3. Ibid.
4. Bennett, K. J. et al. 1987. A controlled trial of teaching critical appraisal of the clinical literature to medical students. *JAMA:* 257(11): 2451.
5. Greenhalgh, T. 1997d. How to read a paper: Papers that summarize other papers (systematic reviews and meta-analyses). *BMJ* 315: 672.
6. Greenhalgh, T. 1997b. How to read a paper: Getting your bearing (deciding what the paper is about). *BMJ* 315: 243ff.
7. Grimes, D. A. 1986. How can we translate good science into good perinatal care? *Birth* 13: 2.
8. Alexander, J. M. et al. 1992. Randomized controlled trial of breast shells and Hoffman's exercises for inverted and non-protractile nipples. *BMJ* 304: 1030.
9. Lawrence, R. A., and R. M. Lawrence. 1999. *Breastfeeding: A Guide for the Medical Profession.* St. Louis, MO: Mosby. 922.
10. Ibid., 255.
11. LACTNET at http://peach.ease.lsoft.com/archives/lactnet.html. (INTERNET.)
12. Rosier, W. 1988. Cool cabbage compresses. *Breastfeeding Rev.* 12: 28–30.
13. Nikodem V. C. et al. 1993. Do cabbage leaves prevent breast engorgement? A randomized, controlled study. *Birth* 20(2): 61.
14. Ibid., 63.
15. Roberts, K. L. et al. 1995b. A comparison of chilled and room temperature cabbage leaves in treating breast engorgement. *J. Hum. Lact.* 11(3): 191.
16. Roberts K. L. et al. 1998. Effects of cabbage leaf extract on breast engorgement. *J. Hum. Lact.* 14: 234.
17. Ibid., 235.
18. Snowden, H. M. et al. 2001. Treatments for breast engorgement during lactation (Cochrane Review) The Cochrane Library. Update Software Ltd. Issue 3.
19. Roberts, K. L. et al. 1998. 125.
20. Beuchat, L. R., and J. H. Ryu. 1997. Produce handling and processing practices. *Emerging Infectious Diseases.* 3(4). Accessed on 9/1/01 at http://www.cdc.gov/ncidod/eid/vol3no4/beuchat.htm (INTERNET).

CHAPTER SEVEN

DEFINING BREASTFEEDING
IN RESEARCH

Charles M. Cadwell, Ph.D.

Introduction

The question of how to define "breastfeeding" has stirred discussion and comment for many years among researchers, policy makers, and program planners.[1] Breastfeeding has been defined as one feeding per day of breast milk for purposes of the mother's inclusion in the Women, Infants, and Children (WIC) program. It has even been described in research as the mother's intent during pregnancy to breastfeed.[2] In general, *any* breastfeeding is totaled in the breastfeeding column, especially in formula company estimates of U.S. breastfeeding rates.[3] This includes all breastfeeding and some breastfeeding, while exclusive formula alone is totaled in the formula column. Sorting through the definitions has resulted in a variety of definitional proposals with the most recognizable related to teaching about Lactational Amenorrhea Method (LAM).[4]

The value of breastfeeding to society in general and the health care system in particular may come down to dollars saved, in spite of other less-measured advantages such as bonding. Third-party payers want to know how much money is to be saved by promoting, protecting, and supporting breastfeeding.[5,6,7] Not every study, though, shows the desired health outcome related to breastfeeding. Could the differences in outcome be due to how breastfeeding was defined in the study by the

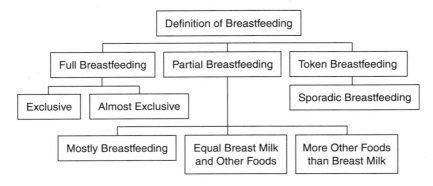

FIGURE 7.1   Schema for breastfeeding definition
Labbok, M. et al. 1994. Guidelines: Breastfeeding, family planning and the Lactational
Amenorrhea Method—LAM. Washington, DC: Institute for Reproductive Health,
Georgetown University.

researchers? One study, for example, defined breastfeeding as "if he or
she was breastfed greater than or equal to 2 times a day, regardless of
other food intakes . . . for one of the two months of the analysis period."[8] The outcome studied was incidence of diarrhea; no significant
difference was found in diarrhea rates between "breastfed" and non-
breastfed infants!

Combinational Analysis

Combinational analysis,[9] a research synthesis methodology that integrates quantitative and qualitative research studies, and responds to the
concern in modern medicine that scientists tend to believe only what
can be measured and observed, even though what can be quantified
may not be what is most important.[10] The combinational analysis
methodology creates a body of knowledge that emerges from the examination of research studies that have investigated a particular area
of interest over a period of time, such as breastfeeding definitions and
health outcomes.

   This chapter includes the results of a combinational analysis by the
author which examines how researchers define breastfeeding and
breastfeeding duration in published studies with a health outcome. One
hundred eighty-six published research studies were examined for the
consistency of definitions of breastfeeding and duration of breastfeeding. Those studies with measured health outcomes as the independent
variables were included in the further analysis. Eighty-four articles

were quantitative research studies in which at least one dependent variable reached statistical significance. Forty-four articles were quantitative research studies in which no statistical significance was found. In 58 of the studies—although breastfeeding benefits appeared either in their title or abstract—were commentaries about ongoing research or quantitative research where conclusions based on breastfeeding were not included in the published study. These 58 were not included in the combinational analysis. The remaining 128 research studies (those that reached significance and those that did not) were examined in the combinational analysis.

The questions asked in the analysis included:

- What definition of breastfeeding, if any, was included in the report of the research studies?
- How was duration of breastfeeding defined and described in the studies?
- How did the definition and/or duration of breastfeeding in studies that examined the same or similar dependent variable differ among studies that had a significant result?
- How did the definition and/or duration of breastfeeding in studies that examined the same or similar dependent variable differ between those studies in which results reached significance and those that did not?
- Is it necessary for future research to include more accurate definitions of breastfeeding and its duration in research studies?

Definitions of Breastfeeding: Statistical Significance Achieved

Eighty-four of the 128 published research studies (65.6 percent) included at least one health outcome in which statistical significance was achieved. Refer to Table 7.1 for a summary. Of the 84 research studies that included at least one case of statistical significance, 34 defined mothers' feeding method as breastfeeding exclusively. Some were worded differently, such as "full breastfeeding," "exclusive breastmilk," or "only breastmilk from mom." This group comprised 40.5 percent of the 84 studies. The next largest group did not define breastfeeding at all. The researcher indicated that the mother "breastfed" or the baby was given "human milk." It is unclear as to whether this is exclusive breastfeeding or a combination of breastfeeding and something else. In 8 studies the author defined breastfeeding as exclusive breastfeeding and something else, such as water, solids, tea, or any combination of these. In defining breastfeeding as "predominantly or exclusively breastfeeding" or "tried to exclusively breastfeed," what other foods were given to the baby? The same question applies to definitions

TABLE 7.1 Definitions of Breastfeeding in Published Research Studies
84 studies that included at least one case of statistical significance

Breastfeeding	Number of Studies	
full breastfeeding	1	(1.2%)
exclusive breastfeeding	27	(32.1%)
exclusive breast milk	5	(6.0%)
only breast milk from mother	1	(1.2%)
	34	**(40.5%)**
exclusive breastfeeding + water	5	(6.0%)
exclusive human milk or human milk + solids	1	(1.2%)
predominantly or exclusively breastfeeding	1	(1.2%)
try exclusive breastfeeding	1	(1.2%)
	8	**(9.5%)**
chose to breastfeed	1	(1.2%)
initiated breastfeeding	1	(1.2%)
encouraged to breastfeed	1	(1.2%)
breastfed at all	2	(2.4%)
any breast milk	2	(2.4%)
any breastfeeding	1	(1.2%)
breastfed + tea + water	3	(3.6%)
no cow's milk or food from cow's milk (soy OK).	3	(3.6%)
breastfed + formula/juices + solids	3	(3.6%)
mixed feeding (breastfed + cow's milk/formula)	2	(2.4%)
	19	**(22.6%)**
human milk (no definition)	2	(2.4%)
breastfed (no definition)	21	(25.0%)
	23	**(27.4%)**

including phrases such as "the mother chose to breastfeed," "initiated breastfeeding," "was encouraged to breastfeed," "breastfed at all," or gave "any breastmilk" to the baby. In some cases breastfeeding was defined in terms of what the baby did not ingest, such as "no cow's milk" or "no food from cow's milk (but that soy was "OK"). Others defined breastfeeding as "breastfed and formula," or "breastfeeding and juices," "breastfeeding and solids," or some combination of breastfeeding, formula, juices, and solids. One defined breastfeeding as "mixed feeding" (breast milk and cow's milk or formula).

In the studies that clearly stated breastfeeding was exclusive, with no other liquids or foods of any kind, one may read the results of the research with greater confidence that breastfeeding may have contributed to some significant conclusion. However, if a researcher defines breastfeeding ambiguously, the reader cannot be convinced that breastfeeding contributed to the conclusion.

TABLE 7.2   Definitions of Breastfeeding in Published Research Studies
44 studies that failed to reach statistical significance

Breastfeeding	Number of Studies	
human milk (no definition)	4	(9.1%)
breastfed (not defined)	15	(34.1%)
breast milk (not defined)	2	(4.5%)
	21	**(47.7%)**
exclusive breastfeeding	16	(36.4%)
exclusive breastfeeding vs. breastfed	1	(2.3%)
exclusive breast milk	1	(2.3%)
	18	**(41.0%)**
exclusive breastfeeding + water	1	(2.3%)
encouraged to breastfeed exclusively	1	(2.3%)
breastfed at all	1	(2.3%)
breastfeeding at least one week and no more than one bottle feeding a day	1	(2.3%)
advised to avoid cow milk foods	1	(2.3%)
	5	**(11.5%)**

Definitions of Breastfeeding: Statistical Significance not Achieved

Forty-four of the 128 published research studies (34.4 percent) failed to reach statistical significance for any health outcome examined. Refer to Table 7.2 for a summary. Studies reaching statistical significance were published at least two times more than those not reaching significance. This fact may be due to publishing companies' preference to report studies with significant statistical outcomes. Of the 44 studies, 19 (43.2%) defined the feeding method as "breastfeed exclusively," with one baby also given water. Twenty-one (47.5 percent) of the studies defined the method as " the mothers breastfed" (where breastfeeding was not defined within the content of the published study). The last four feeding methods were defined as "encouraged to breastfeed," " breastfed at all," "breastfed at least one week and no more than one bottle feeding a day," or "advised to avoid cow milk foods."

Duration of Breastfeeding: Statistical Significance Achieved

The American Academy of Pediatrics recommends that babies be breastfed exclusively for the first six months of life, continuing to the age of one year with the addition of other foods, and then to continue even beyond one year. Of the 84 studies in which at least one health outcome reached statistical significance, only seven studies (8.3 percent) clearly indicated that the breastfeeding mothers breastfed at all

TABLE 7.3   Duration of Breastfeeding in Published Research Studies
84 studies that included at least one case of statistical significance

Duration	Number of Studies	
not defined	28	(33.3%)
	28	**(33.3%)**
any breastfeeding	2	(2.4%)
initiated breastfeeding	1	(1.2%)
	3	**(3.6%)**
first few days	1	(1.2%)
first 4 days	1	(1.2%)
	2	**(2.4%)**
1–20 months	2	(2.4%)
3 months	1	(1.2%)
204 days	1	(1.2%)
5–6 months	2	(2.4%)
	6	**(7.1%)**
≤ 4 months	1	(1.2%)
≤ 6 months	4	(4.8%)
≤ 8 months	1	(1.2%)
≤ 18 months (median 4 months)	1	(1.2%)
	7	**(8.3%)**
≥ 1 month	2	(2.4%)
≥ 1½ months	4	(4.8%)
≥ 2 months	7	(8.3%)
≥ 3 months	5	(6.0%)
≥ 4 months	12	(14.3%)
≥ 5 months	2	(2.4%)
≥ 6 months	6	(7.2%)
	38	**(45.2%)**

for at least six months. See Table 7.3 for a summary. Of the studies, 33.3 percent did not include any information as to the duration of breastfeeding in the study. The remaining portion varied greatly, from "any breastfeeding" and "the first few days" to "more than" a certain month or "less than" a certain month.

Duration of Breastfeeding: Statistical Significance not Achieved

Of the 44 studies where no health outcome reached statistical significance, five studies (11.4 percent) clearly indicated that the breastfeeding mothers breastfed for at least six months. See Table 7.4. Sixteen studies (36.4 percent) did not include any information as to the duration of breastfeeding in the study. The remaining studies also varied greatly, from "any breastfeeding" and "the first few days" to "more than" a certain month or "less than" a certain month.

TABLE 7.4   Duration of Breastfeeding in Published Research Studies
44 studies that failed to reach statistical significance

Duration	Number of Studies	
not defined	16	(36.4%)
	16	**(36.4%)**
any breastfeeding	3	(6.8%)
	3	**(6.8%)**
continued to breastfeed	1	(2.3%)
until introduction of cow's milk or formula	1	(2.3%)
varied	1	(2.3%)
	3	**(6.8%)**
first few days	2	(4.5%)
first 3 days	1	(2.3%)
first 4 days	1	(2.3%)
8 days	1	(2.3%)
first few weeks	1	(2.3%)
2–17 weeks	1	(2.3%)
3–18 months	1	(2.3%)
8 months	1	(2.3%)
15 months	2	(4.5%)
	11	**(25.0%)**
$\leq$ 6 months	1	(2.3%)
	1	**(2.3%)**
$\geq$ 25 days	2	(4.5%)
$\geq$ 1 month	1	(2.3%)
1½ months	1	(2.3%)
$\geq$ 2 months	1	(2.3%)
$\geq$ 3 months	3	(6.8%)
$\geq$ 6 months	1	(2.3%)
$\geq$ 9 months	1	(2.3%)
	10	**(22.8%)**

Definition of Breastfeeding: Comparing the Two Study Groups

The most remarkable difference between these two groups is the percentage of studies in each group that did not define breastfeeding. Refer to Table 7.5. In the group of 23 studies reaching statistical significance, words used to describe the method of feeding the infant were "breast-fed" and "human milk." No further explanation was included. In the group failing to reach significance, words used to describe the method of feeding the infant were "human milk," "breastfed," and "breastmilk," and no further explanation was included in the 21 studies. Comparing the two groups, as a percentage, breastfeeding was not defined in nearly twice the number of studies in the group that failed to reach significance. Likewise, as a percentage, there were close to two and one-half times more studies in the group that reached significance where

TABLE 7.5   Definition of Breastfeeding by Comparing the Study Groups

Group of 84 Reaching Significance:	Group of 44 Failing to Reach Significance:
Exclusive breastfeeding(40.1%)	Exclusive breastfeeding (41.0%)
Exclusive breastfeeding and water (6.0%)	Exclusive breastfeeding and water (2.3%)
Partial breastfeeding (23.7%)	Partial breastfeeding (9.2%)
No definition of breastfeeding (27.4%)	No definition of breastfeeding (47.7%)

TABLE 7.6   Duration of Breastfeeding by Comparing the Study Groups

Group of 84 Reaching Significance:	Group of 44 Failing to Reach Significance:
Breastfeeding duration not defined (33.3%)	Breastfeeding duration not defined (36.4%)
Breastfed less than a month (2.4%)	Breastfed less than a month (13.8%)
Breastfed 3 months or more (36%)	Breastfed 3 months or more (18.4%)
Breastfed 6 months or more (8.3%)	Breastfed 6 months or more (11.5%)

partial breastfeeding occurred. Any attempt to determine correlations is thwarted when breastfeeding is not defined or partially defined in the article. No definition could range from "exclusive breastfeeding" to "intend to breastfeed." "Encouraged to breastfeed" could mean the mother breastfed exclusively or did not breastfeed at all. Thus, comparisons, extrapolations, and conclusions become meaningless.

The Duration of Breastfeeding: Comparing the Two Study Groups

As a percentage, about twice the number of studies where statistical significance occurred had babies breastfeeding for three months or more compared to the group failing to reach significance. Refer to Table 7.6. Similarly, far fewer babies, about one-sixth, breastfed less than one month for the significance group.

Conclusion

Definitions of breastfeeding exclusivity and duration may be related to findings of significance in studies of the relationship between health outcome and breastfeeding. Increased clarity about the value of breastfeeding to society, in general, and to the health care system, in particular, will emerge from attention to definition.

References

1. Labbok, M., and K. Krasovec. 1990. Toward consistency in breastfeeding definitions. *Studies in Family Planning.* 21(4): 226.
2. Paine, R. Jan 1982. Breastfeeding and infant health in a rural U.S. community. *Am. J. Dis. Child.* 136: 36.
3. Martinez, G., and F. Krieger. 1985. Milk feeding patterns in the U.S. *Ped.* 76: 1004.
4. Labbok, M. et al. 1994. Guidelines: Breastfeeding, family planning, and the Lactational Amenorrhea Method—LAM. Washington, DC: Institute for Reproductive Health, Georgetown University.
5. Ball, T. M., and A. L. Wright. 1999. Health care costs of formula feeding in the first year of life. *Pediatrics* 103(4): 870.
6. Tully, J., and K. G. Dewey. Private fears, global loss: A cross-cultural study of the insufficient milk syndrome. *Med. Anthropology* 9: 225.
7. Weimer, J. March 2001. *Economic benefits of breastfeeding.* Report No. 13. *Food Assistance and Nutrition Research. Food and Rural Economics Division,* Economic Research Service, U.S. Department of Agriculture.
8. Cushing, A. December 1982. Diarrhea in breastfed and non breastfed infants. *Peds.* 70(6): 921.
9. Cadwell, C. M., 1995. *Combinational analysis: A model for the synthesis of research studies in behavioral medicine,* University of Michigan.
10. Ornish, D. 1990. *Reversing Heart Disease: The Only System Scientifically Proven to Reverse Heart Disease Without Drugs or Surgery.* New York: Ballantine Books.

CHAPTER EIGHT

PERSONAL MOTIVATIONS FOR BREASTFEEDING

Cindy Turner-Maffei, M.A., I.B.C.L.C., and
Karin Cadwell, Ph.D., R.N., I.B.C.L.C.

As the scientific evidence regarding the benefits of breastfeeding to mother, baby, family, and society mounted during the late twentieth century, the breastfeeding rate floundered. This paradox has troubled many individuals and organizations working to improve maternal child health. Researchers, health care providers, and policy makers have searched for clues to the mystery of breastfeeding initiation and duration. How, when, and why do mothers choose between breast- and formula feeding? What role does education play in assisting choice? Are mothers who succeed at breastfeeding somehow different from mothers who choose formula? How can health care providers best encourage women to consider breastfeeding and to continue breastfeeding once they have begun?

Multiple studies have examined the characteristics of breastfeeding and formula-feeding mothers with diverse findings. In this chapter, the issue of how to support the choice and continuation of breastfeeding will be explored.

Learning to Breastfeed

Breastfeeding is a learned behavior, moderated both by biology and social learning. It is not a purely instinctive behavior.[1] Throughout history women learned how to breastfeed their babies by observing their own lactating mothers, aunts, other clanswomen, and peers. This learning method has changed radically in the past century, as the infant feeding method of the mainstream American culture shifted toward formula. Few women born in the mid to late twentieth century America grew up observing breastfeeding family members; many reached adulthood without ever seeing a baby fed at the breast. As the U.S. breastfeeding rates declined, so did the body of women's breastfeeding knowledge and lore. Many childbearing women today may be the first family members in two or three generations to breastfeed.

Doula and Antidoula

One solution to the breastfeeding success mystery was proposed by Raphael, who, working from an anthropological perspective, noted that it is usual for one or more female members of a traditional society to make themselves available to the mother as an assistant during pregnancy, childbirth, and the neonatal period.[2] This person is usually not a trained midwife but rather a member of the woman's intimate social group; an aunt, mother, or sibling may serve in this role.[3] Acknowledging that a word did not exist in English to describe this relationship, Raphael adopted the ancient Greek word *doula,* meaning female assistant. The doula provides ongoing information, support, and "mothers the mother." Raphael notes that in some cultures, childbearing-age women already knew a considerable amount about breastfeeding because they saw women nursing from the time they were children and also were assured of knowledgable, supportive help during the prenatal time period.[4]

What is in evidence in modern Western cultures can best be described as the antidoula effect. According to Raphael and Jelliffe, not only does a typical new mother have no exposure to breastfeeding as a child, she also is separated geographically from her nuclear family, exposed to unhelpful routines and policies in the hospital, and returned prematurely to nonbaby-focused responsibilities.[5] The failure of breastfeeding in the United States, according to Raphael and Jelliffe can be ascribed to these anti*doula* effects.

Other Factors Influencing the Choice to Breastfeed

From a public health perspective, it is clear that breastfeeding has a positive impact on maternal, child, and societal health. Yet, there is much information in popular culture that distracts from and interferes with the goal of breastfeeding. Women who choose breastfeeding often have to fight against societal conventions and negative input to meet their personal breastfeeding goals. Influenced by a majority culture that is less than supportive of breastfeeding mothers, family members and peers may discourage women from breastfeeding based on stories of pain and embarrassment, coupled with fears about the insufficient milk and inadequate breasts. How can we best encourage women to initiate breastfeeding and support them for its duration? No one answer exists to this puzzle; myriad factors influence women and multiple strategies for success are needed.

A recent thought about the lack of success at breastfeeding in the United States is that there must be some definable quality about the woman herself that compels her to choose breastfeeding for her child and that some quality about the woman determines her breastfeeding success.

In an effort to better understand breastfeeding incidence, Jacobson and colleagues examined *cognitive and personality aspects* of two groups of women: 137 African American inner-city mothers and 50 Caucasian mothers. Breastfeeding rates in the Caucasian mothers were more than twice as high (58 percent vs. 21.9 percent). Researchers found that although breastfeeding was unrelated to maternal depression and social support, it was positively associated with ego maturity and cognitive ability in both samples. Women with more ego maturity may breastfeed because of increased feelings of empathy or nurturance or because they are attuned to current health advisories and able to deviate from community norms to adopt breastfeeding.[6]

> Human lactation is sensitive to a wide variety of interrelated psychological factors, which may be roughly grouped as follows: individual emotions and attitudes; and psychophysiological mediating mechanisms.[7]

Self-Confidence and Breastfeeding[8]

Some researchers have asked whether a woman's degree of *self-confidence* determines the likelihood of her breastfeeding success. Niles Newton tested the power of a mother's attitude in a study of 91 women who chose breastfeeding, finding that mothers who were determined to breastfeed were more likely to be successful. Newton found that 74 percent of mothers who expressed a determination to breastfeed had an adequate milk supply. However, of those mothers who felt that feeding method did not matter, only 35 percent felt they had an "adequate" milk supply.[9] The degree of determination and confidence related to breastfeeding has been associated in this and other studies with successful breastfeeding.[10]

Not every research study has found psychosocial correlates to breastfeeding initiation and duration. Holt and Wolkind found that "few social or psychological variables related to the duration of breast-feeding, nor was there a relationship between the child's temperament and the type of feeding or duration of breastfeeding."[11]

Wagner and Wagner examined the association of maternal attitudes, beliefs, and personality factors with infant feeding choices. They found that maternal attitudes were most predictive of feeding behavior. Women who initiated breastfeeding scored higher on four out of five domains: extraversion, openness, agreeableness, and conscientiousness. These researchers introduced the interesting caveat that retrospective examination of the personality characteristics related to feeding choice is potentially confounded by the changes breastfeeding effects in women's bodies. "The breastfeeding mother is different from the artificially feeding mother in a number of ways. The physical experience of breastfeeding, the hormonal changes following delivery and with sustained breastfeeding, and the emotional aspects are a few of the differences. . . . Personality differences may arise from the physiologic effects of breastfeeding."[12]

Üvnas-Moberg and colleagues made an extensive study of the role of oxytocin on behavior of breastfeeding mothers, concluding that "it is now well established that oxytocin, as well as stimulating uterine contractions and milk ejection, promotes the development of maternal behaviour and also bonding between the mother and offspring."[13] An earlier study from this group found that mothers under the influence of the hormones of lactation are less anxious and more patient than matched controls who were not pregnant or breastfeeding.[14] Thus, examination of personality differences between women during the postpartum period should identify this potential confounding factor and attempt to measure maternal attitudes and characteristics prior to or during pregnancy.

Influence of Support in Choosing Breastfeeding

Socialization is a nearly inextricable factor of individual attitudes. Women's attitudes and intentions toward breastfeeding are influenced by lifelong socialization. Social constructs such as the appropriate role of women of different classes and educational background and the popular image of mothering and breastfeeding influence women's attitudes about breastfeeding. The attitudes of members of women's social support network are likely to have some impact on their feeding choices.

In the late twentieth century, the breastfeeding rates of low-income women were lower than their peers with high incomes. Earlier in the same century, though, the opposite was true: more low-income women were breastfeeding. Mohrer assessed the attitudes and influences on feeding choice of the urban poor and found that women who chose breastfeeding were "generally older, better educated and report living with a male more than other bottle feeders."[15] An examination of the predictors of duration of breastfeeding among low-income women also indicated that the level of education of the mother was a factor.[16] Biegelson and colleagues also documented the low rate of breastfeeding in a low-income population in New York City.[17] Houston and colleagues found similar results in Great Britain: "the association of successful breastfeeding with social class is unclear."[18]

Grossman and colleagues undertook a research study of Ohio women and their infant feeding choices. As the researchers explain, "few studies have described the woman who chooses breastfeeding by more than simple demographics. Age, education, race and socio-economic status are commonly investigated."[19] The Grossman study differed from previous work because in addition to demographics, patterns of support were also examined. Findings were that

> Breastfeeding women were more likely to be older, more educated, married, more affluent, experienced with breastfeeding, to have demonstrated good prenatal habits and to have received support from other sources than those who chose bottle feeding. Participation in Lamaze classes, previous successful breastfeeding, and maternal education were significant predictors of feeding choice. . . . Low income women who chose breastfeeding resembled low income bottle feeders in certain medical/social factors, but they showed support pattern similar to middle income women. . . .[19]
>   . . . More support aimed at encouraging nursing is needed from professionals, family members and friends and possibly through "mother to mother" counseling from La Leche League or similar groups for low income pregnant women who have never successfully nursed, who have little education, and who do not wish to attend prenatal childbirth classes.[20]

This research, then, may be said to reframe the breastfeeding success outcome to one in which the pattern of support becomes a definable quality in the woman who chooses to breastfeed.

Several researchers have also explored the role played by the attitudes of the father of the baby and other significant family members in determining breastfeeding behavior.[21] Littman and colleagues found that the father's level of education and his degree of approval for breastfeeding were the only factors examined that were linked with initiation of breastfeeding in their study population: 98.1 percent of women who initiated breastfeeding had partners who strongly approved of breastfeeding, but the indifferent attitude of other fathers toward breastfeeding was associated with a 26.9 percent initiation rate.[22] In a pilot survey conducted in 12 Missouri WIC program agencies, researchers found that the main support for women choosing to breastfeed came from their husbands.[23] However, Giugliani and colleagues, surveying fathers in Baltimore, found that fathers had poor knowledge of breastfeeding.[24]

The identity of most influential social network members varies among ethnic cultures and among individual women. Among population groups studied in Florida, only Anglo women expected support from the babies' fathers.[25] In other cultures, it was the mothers' mother, sister, or health care provider whose opinion was most influential in their decision making.[26] Wagner and Wagner found that the feeding preference of the babies' maternal grandmother, was significantly correlated with the breastfeeding choice of the babies' mother. Of the grandmothers who preferred breastfeeding, 87 percent of their daughters chose breastfeeding; of those grandmothers who preferred formula, only 16 percent of their daughters chose breastfeeding.[27] For other women, friends may be the most powerful influence. Entwisle and colleagues found that a woman's persistence at breastfeeding was correlated with the breastfeeding success among her female friends.[28] While health care providers have been found to have some influence on breastfeeding initiation, friends and family have been found to be more influential than health care providers.[29]

Summarizing the importance of reaching out to social support networks, Losch and colleagues write:

> It is not sufficient for . . . programs to target only the mother or potential mother; members of a woman's social support network must be considered as information targets. Educational programs must also be directed to the appropriate racial or ethnic group to develop programs that reach the individuals (father, female relatives, or friend) most likely to influence the mother's breast-feeding decision.[30]

Factors Impacting Duration of Breastfeeding

It is crucial to understand what encourages women to continue breastfeeding in order to ensure breastfeeding duration. In many American communities, the majority of women attempt breastfeeding, but few reach the Healthy People 2010 targets for duration at six and twelve months. In fact, few women reach their own stated goals for duration. One of the most common reasons given for discontinuing breastfeeding before the intended weaning age is the mother's fear that she does not have enough milk. This is also a common reason for the introduction of breast milk substitutes and weaning foods before the recommended age of the baby.

Newton and Newton outlined a model for the psychological aspects of lactation as a response to their growing concern for the increase in lactation failure.

> The rapidity with which lactation failure spreads through human groups suggests that it is triggered by psychological factors. For instance, national surveys indicate that the neonatal breast-feeding rate in the United States fell by almost half during just ten years. In the course of twenty years in Bristol, England, the number of three-month-old breast-fed infants dropped from 77 to 36 percent. In an obstetric clinic in France the proportion of babies getting no breast milk increased from 31 to 51 percent in just five years. This decrease is so rapid that hereditary factors could not be operative and major physiological changes in function would be unlikely in the absence of radical stresses such as starvation or epidemic disease. Human emotions and behavior, however, may change rapidly in keeping with the rapid changes observed in rates of breastfeeding.[31]

Segura-Millan and colleagues found that 80 percent of the women reported at least one occasion of perceived insufficient milk.[32] Gussler and Briesemeister coined the phrase "insufficient milk syndrome" (IMS) to indicate that there is no single cause for the problem; indeed it is a complex relation of biological, sociological, psychological, cultural, and political factors that play into the concern about milk supply.

> One of the most difficult situations involves the mother who thinks that she does not have enough milk and makes changes in her life that she erroneously believes will increase her milk supply. She may, for example, decrease the number of feedings per day in the mistaken belief that this will rest the breasts so they will increase milk production. Or, she may decrease the number of feeds per day, believing that her milk will 'store up' and feel full. She mistakenly believes that this will increase the milk she gives at each feed so that the baby will be more satisfied. Unfortunately, spacing out feeding decreases, rather than increases, the quantity of milk.[33]

Neifert and Seacat have described maternal and infant factors that may be associated with impaired lactation. These include: breast surgery that damaged lactiferous ducts, nipple innervation, and infants with an inadequate suck. The authors conclude,

> The challenge for the health professional is to distinguish primary, nonremediable etiologies of insufficient lactation from secondary management problems, and to institute appropriate early intervention. The aim is to preserve the breastfeeding relationship where desired and to achieve maximum potential milk supply where possible, without ever jeopardizing an infant's nutritional well-being.[34]

One might naively think that a fussy baby is a hungry baby and a quiet baby is a full and content baby. Within the range of "normal" this may hold true, but underfed, calorically deprived babies begin to conserve energy, cry less, and sleep more. Unfortunately, this behavior, on the part of the baby may serve to reinforce the mother's behavior of restricting feeds. As the baby continues to be calorically deprived, the suck may weaken, further diminishing the stimulus required by the mother's breasts to continue producing an adequate supply of milk. This example demonstrates how a mother with an adequate milk supply may diminish her quantity of milk by unfortunate behavior intended to increase her milk supply.

Tully and Dewey studied the feeding practices of four ethnic groups in the Davis-Sacramento area of California and in Kingston, Jamaica. The four groups represented were Anglo-Americans, Mexican-Americans, Mexican-born, and Jamaican. The authors report that 35–40 percent of the mothers in all four ethnic groups reported insufficient milk within the first six weeks. They state:

> The cue that prompted mothers to believe their milk was insufficient in most cases was that the baby cried or did not appear satisfied after nursing. 'Breasts did not feel full' was the second most commonly cited reason among all except Mexican-Americans. A few mothers in all groups except the Anglos stated there was no evidence of milk coming from the breast.[35]

The authors continue, "The most common response to insufficient milk was the introduction of a supplementary bottle. Mexican-born mothers were the most likely to introduce a bottle, while Anglos were least likely to do so."[36]

Tully and Dewey delineate three factors significantly associated with insufficient milk syndrome:

- Low infant birth weight
- Provision of formula in the hospital
- Maternal attitude that breastfeeding is "inconvenient"[37]

> The greater frequency of IMS among mothers who felt that breastfeeding is "inconvenient" suggests a psychosocial basis for IMS. In the current study, mothers who described breastfeeding as inconvenient were also more likely to introduce a supplementary bottle, which may have been the intermediary factor between maternal attitude and IMS. However, it is unclear in these cases whether the bottle is antecedent to or followed the perception of insufficient milk.[38]

In a prospective study in Colorado, Demarzo and colleagues followed 125 motivated, primiparous women from the third trimester of pregnancy. Participating women were required to attend a prenatal breastfeeding class and have their breasts examined prenatally. They were seen by the clinician at four to seven and nine to fourteen days postpartum and were given access to a lactation clinician via phone or pager. Mothers recorded feeding and elimination data. Infant weight was recorded at each visit on an electronic scale, and test weights to assess milk intake were also performed at each visit. All detected breastfeeding problems, including engorgement, suckling problems, and sore nipples were treated promptly.[39] Researchers found that 6.4 percent[38] of women participating in the study had persistent, inadequate lactation, "despite high motivation, ready access to counseling, early follow-up and aggressive intervention for secondary difficulties."[40]

Houston, on the other hand, was able to constitute an intervention that eliminated the problem of insufficient milk in a population of women in Great Britain. The mothers in the study group received home visits. As much as possible, continuity of care was provided by having the same person, a midwife, visit the mother each time.[41]

> At each visit the baby's pattern of feeding was discussed, together with problems which the mother mentioned. Mothers were encouraged to make their own decisions regarding the continuation of feeding. . . .[42]
>
> . . . Mothers in the study group (the home visit group) introduced supplementary food, in the form of formula milk or solids, significantly later than mothers in the control group. In all social classes, [they] were more confident in their ability fully to breast feed their baby. It was notable that none of the study group stopped due to "insufficient milk" in contrast to (15%) mothers in the control group.[43]

One of the critical issues surrounding the insufficient milk syndrome for clinicians who manage lactation care and for breastfeeding specialists is whether it is a valid or a perceived problem of not enough milk.[44] The case reports of failure to thrive and critical malnutrition in otherwise seemingly healthy breastfed babies appear regularly in the professional literature as well as the lay press and news media.[45] These tragic stories seem remarkably similar. The babies are healthy and born at term to intelligent, motivated mothers.[46] The babies are brought to the physician's attention usually for a problem that seemingly has nothing to do with the mother's worries about her milk supply—a rash or odd bowel movements, for example.[47] These are not babies of mothers who are worried about not having enough milk.[48] Why? Because the babies do not cry, fuss, or act demanding so the mother assumes she has plenty of milk.[49] The babies are grossly malnourished and exhibit abnormal behavior such as sleeping for twenty hours or going nine hours between feedings.

As numerous authors suggest, caloric deprivation decreases the baby's alertness and increases the amount of sleep, thus giving the naive mother the impression she has a contented, adequately nourished baby.[50,51]

Some mothers who perceive that they do not have enough milk may actually have an adequate milk supply. According to Hillervik-Lindquist's work as well as Segura-Millan, the majority of mothers have *perceived* (not actual) milk sufficiency. As described above, access to help and secondary interventions such as breast pumping may have little impact on the problem,[52] while home visits as a primary intervention may.[53] This concept of early intervention or case finding is seldom implemented in the United States.

> **Primary Intervention** (case finding) can include practices such as home visits to all mothers

> **Secondary Interventions** can include practices such as giving mothers access to help and providing support when needed after a problem is discovered

In separate studies, **only primary intervention seems to prevent or decrease breastfeeding failure due to insufficient milk supply.**

References and Notes

1. Ladas, A. K. 1970. How to help mother breastfeed: Deduction from a survey. *Clin. Peds.* 9(12): 702.
2. Raphael, D. 1973. *The tender gift: Breastfeeding.* Englewood Cliffs, NJ: Prentice Hall, Inc.
3. Raphael, D. 1966. The lactation-sucking process within a matrix of social support. Ph.D. thesis, Columbia University.
4. Raphael, D. 1973. The role of breastfeeding in a bottle-oriented world. *Ecol. Fd. Nutr.* 2: 121.
5. Raphael, D., and E. Jelliffe. 1973. Education of the public for successful lactation. *Ecol. Fd. Nutr.* 2: 126.
6. Jacobson, S. et al. 1991. Incidence and correlates of breastfeeding in socioeconomically disadvantaged women. *Peds.* 88(4): 728.
7. Newton, N., and M. Newton. 1967. Psychological Aspects of Lactation. *NEJM.* 227(22): 1179.
8. Jelliffe, D. B., and E. F. P. Jelliffe. 1978. Breast feeding is best for infants everywhere. *Nutr. Today* 1978b(3): 12.
9. Newton, N. 1955. Women's feelings about breast feeding. *Maternal Emotions.* New York: Hoeber. 43ff.
10. Coreil J., and J. Murphy. 1988. Maternal commitment, lactation practices and breastfeeding duration. *J. Obstet. Gynecol. Neonatal Nurs.* 4: 273. Dungy, C. I. et al. 1994. Maternal attitudes as predictors of infant feeding decisions. *J. Assoc. Acad. Minor. Phys.* 5(4): 159.

Entwisle, D. R. et al. 1982. Sociopsychological determinants of women's breastfeeding behavior. *Am. J. Orthopsychiatry* 52: 244.

11. Holt, G., and S. Wolkind. 1983. Early abandonment of breastfeeding: Causes and effects. *Child: Care, Health and Devel.* 9: 349.

12. Wagner, C. L., and M. T. Wagner. 1999. The breast or the bottle? Determinants of infant feeding behaviors. *Clin. Perinatol* 26(2): 505.

13. Üvnas-Moberg, K., and M. Eriksson. 1996 Breastfeeding: physiological, endocrine and behavioural adaptations caused by oxytocin and local neurogenic activity in the nipple. *Acta Pediatr Scand* 85: 525.

14. Üvnas-Moberg, K. et al. 1990. Personality traits in women 4 days postpartum and their correlation with plasma levels of oxytocin and prolactin. *J. Psychosom. Obstet. Gynecol.* 11: 261.

15. Mohrer, J. 1979. Breast and bottle feeding among the urban poor: An assessment of influences, attitudes and practices. *Med. Anthro.* 79: 125.

16. Hawkins, L. et al. 1987. Predictors of the duration of breastfeeding on low-income women. *Birth* 14(4): 204.

17. Biegelson, D. 1986 Breastfeeding practices in a low income population in New York City: a study of selected health department and child health stations. *J Am Diet Assoc.* 86(1): 90.

18. Houston, M. et al. 1983. Factors affecting the duration of breastfeeding: 2 Early feeding practices and social class. *Early Hum. Dev.* 8(1): 55.

19. Grossman, L. et al. 1990. The infant feeding decision in low and upper income women. *Clin. Peds.* 29(1): 30.

20. Grossman, L. et al. 1990. 36–37.

21. Libbus, M. K., and L. S. Kolostov. 1994. Perceptions of breastfeeding and infant feeding choice in a group of low-income mid-Missouri women. *J. Hum. Lact.* 10(1): 17.

Matthews, K. et al. 1998. Maternal infant-feeding decisions: Reasons and influences. *Can. J. Nurs. Res.* 30(2): 177.

Scott, J. A., and C. W. Binns. 1999. Factors associated with the initiation and duration of breastfeeding: A review of the literature. *Breastfeeding Rev.* 7(1): 5.

Yeung, D. L. et al. 1981. Breastfeeding: Prevalence and influencing factors. *Can. J. Pub. Health* 72: 323.

Bar-Yam, N. B., and L. Darby. 1997. Fathers and breastfeeding: A review of the literature. *J. Hum. Lact.* 13(1): 45.

Sharma, M., and R. Petosa. 1997. Impact of expectant fathers in breastfeeding decisions. *J. Am. Diet. Assoc.* 97: 1311.

22. Littman, H. et al. 1994. The decision to breastfeed: The importance of father's approval. *Clin. Pediatr.* 33(4): 214.

23. McClurg-Hitt, D., and J. Olsen. 1994. Infant feeding decisions in the Missouri WIC Program. *J Hum Lact* 10: 253.

24. Giugliani, E. R. J. et al. 1994. Are fathers prepared to encourage their partners to breast feed? A study about fathers' knowledge of breast feeding. *Acta. Paediat.* 83: 1127.

25. Bryant, C. A. 1982. Impact of kin, friend and neighbor networks on infant feeding practices. *Soc. Sci. Med.* 17: 57.

26. Martens, P. J. 1997. Prenatal infant feeding intent and perceived social support for breastfeeding in Manitoba first nations communities: A role for health care providers. *Int. J. Circumpolar Health* 56(4): 104.

27. Wagner. C. L., and M. T. Wagner. 1999.

28. Entwisle, D. R. et al. 1982.

29. Lu, M.D. et al. 2001. Provider encouragement of breast-feeding: Evidence from a national survey. *Obstet. Gynecol.* 97(2): 290.
    Ekwo, E. E. et al. 1983. Factors influencing initiation of breast-feeding. *Am. J. Dis. Child.* 137: 375.

30. Losch, M. et al. 1995. Impact of attitudes on maternal decision regarding infant feeding. *J. Pediatr.* 126(4): 507.

31. Newton, N., and M. Newton. 1967.

32. Segura-Millan, S. et al. 1994. Factors associated with perceived insufficient milk in low income populations in Mexico. *J. Nutr.* 124: 202.

33. Gussler, J., and L. Briesemeister. 1980. The insufficient milk syndrome: A biocultural explanation. *Med. Anthro.* 4(2): 145.

34. Neifert, M., and J. Seacat. 1987. Lactation insufficiency: A rational approach. *Birth.* 14(4): 182.

35. Tully, J., and K. Dewey. 1985. Private fears, global loss: A cross-cultural study of the insufficient milk syndrome. *Med. Anthro.* 85: 225, 235.

36. Ibid., 236.

37. Ibid., 240.

38. Ibid., 240–241.

39. Demarzo, S. et al. 1990. A prospective study of the incidence of insufficient lactation despite optimal breastfeeding management. In *Breastfeeding, Nutrition, Infection and Infant Growth in Developed and Emerging Countries.* S. A. Atkinson et al., eds. St. Johns, Newfoundland, Canada: ARTS Biomedical publishers, 519–520.

40. Vahlquist and others have estimated that perhaps 5 to 10 percent of women worldwide are unable to lactate. Vahlquist, B. 1981. *Introduction In Contemporary Patterns of Breast-feeding: Report on WHO Collaborative on Breast-feeding.* Geneva: World Health Organization.

41. Houston, M. 1984. Supporting breast-feeding at home. *Mid. Chron. and Nsg Notes.* February, 42–44.

42. Ibid., 42.

43. Ibid., 43.

44. Segura-Millan, S. et al. 1994. The authors avoid the term "Insufficient Milk Syndrome" (IMS). ". . . (I)n this paper we have purposely avoided the use of the term 'insufficient milk syndrome.' The available evidence from well-nourished and marginally malnourished populations suggests that this condition is neither a disease nor a syndrome in the clinical sense of the word."
    "In conclusion, our results suggest that such public health options as educational messages explaining the process of lactogenesis during the first days after delivery (targeting both mothers and health workers), assisting women with the prevention and treatment of sore nipples and prenatally increasing maternal confidence in breast-feeding could reduce

PIM (Perceiving Insufficient Milk) and therefore improve breast-feeding success and infant well-being."

Hillervik-Lindquist, C. et al. 1991. Studies on Perceived Milk Insufficiency III: Consequences for breast milk consumption and growth. *Acta. Paediatr. Scand.* 80: 297–303. The authors followed 51 mother-infant pairs prospectively for the period three days to eighteen months after delivery, and 54.9 percent of the mothers reported transient lactation crisis of perceived milk insufficiency. ". . . (E)vidence was provided that the breast milk insufficiency occasionally perceived as acute by the mothers was in most cases real" (p. 297).

The determinants of IMS are also discussed in Hill's article "Insufficient Milk Supply Syndrome" in *NAACOG's Clinical Issues,* 1992, 605–612.

45. Gilmore, R., and T. Rowland. 1978. Critical malnutrition in breast-fed infants. *Am. J. Dis. Child.* 132, 885–887. [Article also published in *Wall Street Journal, New York Times,* and *Time Magazine.*]
46. Roddey, O. F. et al. 1981. Critical weight loss and malnutrition in breast-fed infants. *Am. J. Dis. Child.* 135: 597.
47. Rowland, T. et al. 1982. Malnutrition and hypernatremic dehydration in breastfed infants. *J. Am. Med. Assoc.* 247(7): 1016.
48. Rushton, A. et al. 1982. Dehydration in a breast-fed infant (letter) *J. Am. Med. Assoc.* 248: 6646.
49. Grisham, F., and J. Roloff. 1983. Malnutrition and hypernatremic dehydration in two breast-fed infants. *Clin. Ped.* 22(8): 592.
50. Grisham and Roloff, 1983.
51. Gilmore, R., and T. Rowland. 1978, 886.
52. DeMarzo, S. et al. 1990.
53. Hillervik-Lindquist, C. et al. 1991. Houston, M. 1984.

CHAPTER NINE

OVERCOMING DISPARITIES IN BREASTFEEDING

Cindy Turner-Maffei, M.A., I.B.C.L.C.

Disparities in the health of our nation's population are of growing concern. Infant mortality, shorter life expectancy, and cancer are among the negative outcomes unevenly distributed among people of different gender, race, ethnicity, education, income, disability, and geographic location. Healthy People 2010's Goal 2 is to eliminate health disparities.[1]

Racial and Ethnic Factors in Breastfeeding

U.S. Surgeon General and Assistant Secretary for Health David Satcher has sounded the call for overcoming disparities in breastfeeding:

> Low breastfeeding rates documented in the Blueprint for Action are a serious public health challenge, particularly in certain minority communities. . . . With scientific evidence indicating that breastfeeding can play an important role in an infant's health, the time has come for us to work together to promote optimal breastfeeding practices. Each of us, at all levels of the public and private sectors, must now turn these recommendations into programs that best suit the needs of our own communities.[2]

Recent statistics indicate that 64 percent of American mothers breastfeed in the early postpartum period, with 29 percent still breastfeeding six months after birth. Racial and ethnic disparities in breastfeeding are wide, particularly among African American women. See

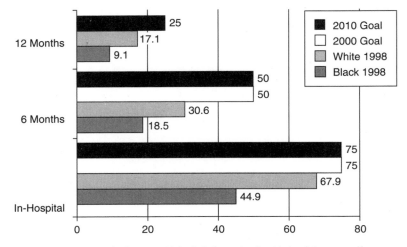

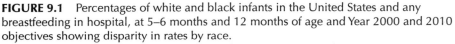

FIGURE 9.1   Percentages of white and black infants in the United States and any breastfeeding in hospital, at 5–6 months and 12 months of age and Year 2000 and 2010 objectives showing disparity in rates by race.
Data from Ross Products Division, Abbott Laboratories Ross Mothers' Survey.

Figure 9.1. In 1998, 45 percent of African American mothers breastfed their infants in the early postpartum period, compared to 66 percent of Hispanic mothers and 68 percent of Caucasian mothers. Only 19 percent of African American mothers continued to breastfeed at six months, compared to 28 percent of Hispanic mothers and 31 percent of Caucasian mothers.[3] That same year, 54 percent of low-income Asian and Pacific Islander women and 59 percent of American Indian and Alaskan Native women initiated breastfeeding.[4] The speculation that infant mortality, as well as morbidity, may be linked to lower rates of breastfeeding in African-American infants is of concern. "By increasing breastfeeding among black women, the racial gap in infant mortality should narrow—a gap that is currently (1997) about 1.3 times higher for blacks than whites."[5]

Economic Factors in Breastfeeding

Family income is associated with disparity in breastfeeding rates. Women who qualify for the federal Special Supplemental Food Program for Women, Infants, and Children (WIC) have low to moderate household income. WIC breastfeeding initiation and duration rates run consistently lower than the general population; the 1997 Ross Mothers' Survey showed that 47 percent of WIC participants initiated

- Slightly over one-half of the WIC mothers initiate breastfeeding.
- Substantial proportions of WIC mothers experience several hospital practices that are unsupportive of the establishment of breastfeeding immediately after birth.
- Less than one-third of WIC infants receive breast milk at their first feeding. Among the infants who ever breastfeed, only a small minority begin breastfeeding during the first hour after birth and only one-half breastfeed during the first three hours.
- During the hospital stay, almost three-fourths of the infants spend at least one night in the nursery away from their mothers.
- Almost one-third of the breastfeeding mothers who experience nursing problems in the hospital do not receive any help from the hospital staff.
- Almost all mothers, including exclusively breastfeeding mothers, receive a hospital gift package that contains a bottle, formula, sugar water, or a pacifier not supportive of breastfeeding.
- About one-half of breastfeeding infants are given formula during the first two weeks of life. One-fourth of breastfeeding infants receive formula by the age of five days.
- One-fourth of the WIC mothers who initiate breastfeeding stop by the end of the second week and one-half stop by the end of the second month postpartum.
- A majority of the breastfeeding WIC mothers experience nursing problems during the first few months.

FIGURE 9.2   Selected Findings of the WIC Infant Feeding Practices Study. *Source:* Adapted from Baydar, N. et al. 1997. WIC Infant Feeding Practices Study: Summary of Findings. Alexandria, VA: United States Department of Agriculture.

breastfeeding, compared with 71 percent of nonparticipants. At that time, six month breastfeeding duration rates were 13 percent among WIC participants and 29 percent among non-WIC participants.[6]

The WIC Infant Feeding Practices Study examined the experience of 987 pregnant and 245 infant WIC participants.[7] The findings pertinent to breastfeeding appear in Figure 9.2.

Geographic Factors in Breastfeeding

Location of residence is an associated factor in breastfeeding. Initiation rates range from a high of 75 percent in the pacific and neighboring mountain regions to a low of 44 percent in the east south central region.[8] This variation underscores the thought that culture, norms, and practices specific to different geographic areas may greatly influence women's choices.

Cultural Factors in Breastfeeding

The value of breastfeeding is not absolute; many people do not believe there is a difference between breast milk and formula. Breastfeeding is a largely invisible activity in the United States.[9] Breastfeeding mothers are rarely observed in public, and there is much negative feeling about the prospect of visible public nursing. Formula and bottles are visible everywhere: on television, in print advertising, in the supermarket, and in or on the diaper bag hanging from every stroller in the shopping mall. For some low-income women, particularly recent immigrants, formula may have greater perceived value than breast milk. Gifts of formula from hospitals, health care providers, and government programs have been associated with declines in breastfeeding initiation, exclusivity, and duration.[10] Formula is one of the only food benefits the federal government provides for the infants of low- to moderate-income families through the WIC program. Regardless of the excellent breastfeeding programs established in most WIC programs, women may perceive that formula is the food the government wishes their babies to receive. Another barrier for many women, particularly those who are low-wage earners, is achieving the degree of workplace accommodation for nursing or milk expression breaks that is attained by higher wage earning cohorts.

The rapidity with which women immigrants adapt to the breastfeeding choices and patterns of a new culture speaks of the power of cultural norms. In a comparison of Turkish mothers who had recently emigrated to Sweden with Turkish mothers in Istanbul, Kocturk and Zetterstrom found that the Turkish women who lived in Stockholm were most likely to nurse and wean in a Swedish pattern rather than a Turkish pattern, showing twenty years later the validity of the Newton's model.[11] Romero-Gwynn described similar findings among Indo-Chinese immigrants in northern California. Before emigration, 94 percent of mothers breastfed exclusively; only 3.8 percent intended to exclusively nurse their new babies in the United States. Romero-Gwynn speculates that there is a miscommunication of recommended feeding practices to immigrant women. Dramatically, 98 percent of a group of Chinese emigrants breastfed their last baby born in China; only 2 percent of the sample chose to breastfeed their first child born in the United Kingdom.[12] Researchers working with immigrants from numerous national origins have theorized that these changes in breastfeeding patterns may reflect women's assimilation of the infant feeding norms of their new nation.[13] Summarizing their work with Mexican Americans, Raissin and colleagues write, "These data support the hypothesis that mothers least acculturated to the United States are most likely to breastfeed. Thus, adaptation to the culture of the United States somehow influences infant-feeding choices."[14]

Cultural beliefs can be barriers to or facilitators of breastfeeding. Traditions, beliefs, and values surrounding breastfeeding vary widely among the world's cultures. In the United States there is a prominent cultural belief that breastfeeding in public is distasteful. Adherence to this belief may cause women to believe that breastfeeding is something that may be done only in the privacy of their own bedrooms.

Colostrum, the first milk produced by the breast, may be a subject of cultural notoriety. In some traditional cultures, breastfeeding is not practiced in the first days of life because colostrum is felt to be unhealthful, or even evil.[15] The practice of feeding an infant other foods, including formula, during the first days of life may lead health care workers to assume erroneously that a mother has chosen not to breastfeed. Rather, she may be waiting to breastfeed until her milk has turned from colostrum to mature milk. The opportunity to have an ongoing dialogue about breastfeeding may be lost if the situation is not clearly understood.

Exploring cultural beliefs is an important step. Summarizing their work with Hmong and Vietnamese mothers, Tuttle and Dewey write ". . . mothers in both groups . . . viewed the convenience and popularity of bottle-feeding as major reasons not to breast-feed. The economic advantages of breastfeeding were not relevant to them because they obtained free formula from WIC, and the health advantages were not obvious to them because they associated breast-feeding with thinness of infants in their native land. . . . The promotion of breast-feeding needs to focus on issues considered important to these women, such as increased time between pregnancies, fewer episodes of specific illnesses for their babies, and convenience."[16]

Who can provide information that challenges cultural beliefs? Can a health care provider convince a woman practicing colostral taboos to feed colostrum to her baby? Statements of authority figures may be received positively or negatively by members of minority culture. Some cultures value authority figures, while others seek authority within. Rejecting medical advice may be perceived as an act of autonomy by some.[17] Breastfeeding promotion campaigns have the potential to be counterproductive if perceived to be authority-based. Programs should be carefully designed with the input of members of the target community.

Racial and ethnic prejudices, real and perceived, of the majority culture influence the activities and choices of members of minority cultures. Several cases of brain damage, extreme dehydration, and (rarely) infant death associated with inadequate breast milk intake have appeared in the media in the past decade. Racial and ethnic prejudices are visible in this coverage as well. A case in point was the intense media coverage of the tragic starvation death of a breastfed African American infant and the subsequent legal action against his mother, Tabitha

Waldron.[18] While Ms. Waldron was indicted and found guilty in the death of her infant, several Caucasian middle-class mothers who experienced similar tragic losses have been heralded as martyrs, rather than criminals. The titles and subtitles of the articles written about the unfortunate Caucasian mothers (" 'Yuppie Syndrome' Among Well-Meaning Parents Stems from Bad Advice"[19] and "When Breast-Feeding Fails: Low-Milk Syndrome Poses a Rare but Frightening Risk")[20] are very different in tone from the Waldron case ("Placing the Blame in an Infant's Death: Mother Faces Trial After Baby Dies from Lack of Breast Milk"[21] and "Bronx Woman Convicted in Starving of Her Breast-Fed Son"[22]). All of the articles mentioned above include photos or artwork that clearly indicate the race of the respective mothers. Understandably, women may conclude that breastfeeding is a dangerous activity, particularly when it might lead to charges of infanticide.

Access to Health Care Services

Access to health care services, including breastfeeding care, may be limited by financial, language, geographic, and cultural barriers. Beyond routine in-hospital care, often breastfeeding services are not provided by clinics or covered by insurers. Lactation care and services may be beyond the means of many families.

Disparities are also noted in content of health care. Kogan and colleagues obtained information from the National Maternal and Infant Health Survey of the advice that health care providers gave 8,310 African American and Caucasian women during prenatal care.

> Advice promoting breast-feeding was the advice reported least often. In general, there was some tendency for women of higher socioeconomic status to get more breast-feeding advice. Breast-feeding advice was more frequent in Whites, married women, and women with more than 12 years of education; it was least frequent in the lowest-income women. Site of prenatal care presents a complex picture, with HMOs and publicly funded clinics the most frequent providers of breast-feeding information. WIC participants reported only a 54.7% rate of receiving breast-feeding advice from their health care providers. . . . The present study suggests that large numbers of women of all races do not receive sufficient health behavior modification information as part of the content of their prenatal care. In particular, Black women are more likely not to receive health behavior advice that could reduce their chances of having an adverse pregnancy outcome.[23]

Other factors that influence breastfeeding include the ease of integrating breastfeeding with employment outside the home.[24] (For a discussion of workplace issues and breastfeeding, see Chapter 10.)

Overcoming Disparities: Limitations of Education

What strategies are helpful in bringing breastfeeding back into the consciousness of women? Breastfeeding advocates often think of education as the ultimate tool. Those who embrace the well-documented health advantages of breastfeeding often assume that the information alone is all it will take to convince women to choose breastfeeding. "We have such excellent data on the benefits of breastfeeding now—all we need to do is to get women to listen to the facts."

Results of researchers looking at the impact of education strategies on breastfeeding have produced mixed results. Shand and Kosawa compared the impact of different information sources on American and Japanese primiparous women.[25] Compared to their Japanese counterparts, American women used a variety of approaches to learning, including formal and informal learning. In this research population hospital classes on breastfeeding were associated with negative breastfeeding trends: women who attended breastfeeding classes were less likely to initiate breastfeeding and more likely to supplement if they chose breastfeeding.

Other researchers have found that carefully targeted breastfeeding education has a positive effect on breastfeeding rates. Kistin and colleagues compared two approaches to breastfeeding education: one-on-one counseling with a health care provider and group classes with a control group receiving no special education.[26] They found that women in both experimental groups were more likely to choose breastfeeding than controls. Those who received individual counseling initiated breastfeeding at a slightly higher rate than those who attended groups. More women who attended the groups subsequently changed their intention from formula feeding to breastfeeding. The researchers note that it is important to explore women's negative perceptions about breastfeeding.

The impetus to promote breastfeeding often devolves into attempts to exert persuasive powers on a single individual who is fully engaged in one of life's most challenging and humbling tasks: becoming a mother. With notable exceptions,[27] American breastfeeding promotion activities and campaigns have been oriented almost exclusively toward education: getting detailed information about the health benefits of breastfeeding directly to individual pregnant women. Breastfeeding promotion may be mistakenly seen as a "bullet" approach; i.e., give women the information and they will perform the desired activity. Such an approach does not address the complex issues that surround the infant feeding decision.

Health behavior change campaigns such as those sponsored by antismoking and antidrug use initiatives have become visible models for those wishing to change other behaviors such as nonbreastfeeding. However, communication scholars have criticized individual health behavior change campaigns for their single-minded focus on the individual's choices without regard for social and environmental factors, as well as for restricting the flow of information so that the target individual is not empowered to interact with the messenger.[28] Interaction provides a forum for the individual to ask questions, explore the meaning message and the ramifications of the behavior, and explore methods to apply the message.

It is difficult to define the factors and strategies that help individuals effect change in their health behaviors. However, it has become clear that education alone is not effective. Information and education may not lead to the intended outcome when other factors stand in the way. "Education is not a sufficient condition for inducing cooperation with medical regimens . . . because much human behavior is not perfectly rational. Among other factors, people are heavily influenced by cultural expectations, by social influence and social support, by self-concept, by pursuit of pleasure and avoidance of difficulties, and even by habit."[29]

In order to choose breastfeeding, individuals need to perceive it as both desirable *and* achievable. Education campaigns alone are unlikely to lead to this double-prong result. For example, nearly every American receives educational messages on a daily basis about the importance of exercise. Every individual knows that exercise is an activity that is beneficial to health; most people would like to be more physically fit. Yet the majority fail to incorporate exercise into daily life, in part because they do not perceive it to be an achievable goal. In order to consider breastfeeding, women need to see and hear that it is feasible to fit breastfeeding into their lives. The majority of breastfeeding stories in current urban mythology involve pain, inadequacy, embarrassment, and humiliation. These themes do not support a cultural image of breastfeeding as desirable and achievable. When interviewed privately, many women tell moving stories about the positive meaning of breastfeeding in their lives. However, it is rare to hear women in public conversations telling their peers stories about their positive breastfeeding experiences. Perhaps the cultural confusion of breastfeeding and sexuality lends these stories a touch of taboo. Yet, in order to move the image of breastfeeding toward desirability and achievability, positive stories need to be heard.

Social Learning

What are the factors standing between acquired knowledge and willingness to apply knowledge? Bandura's social cognitive theory offers some helpful insights. The organizing principle of this theory is *per-*

ceived self-efficacy, defined as "people's beliefs that they can exert control over their motivation and behavior and over their social environment."[30] When choosing whether or not to breastfeed, a woman is not just considering information, but also assessing her own personal power, her physical and emotional capability to surmount the real and imagined barriers standing in the way of her success at breastfeeding. Inundating a woman with education about health benefits of breastfeeding may be counterproductive at a time when she may doubt even her ability to carry her baby to term.

Bryant and colleagues write:

> For interventions to be successful, they must be grounded in research on women's attitudes and needs and on an understanding of the larger social factors that shape women's decisions. Women's misgivings about the feasibility of breastfeeding often are based on incomplete and inaccurate information. Women's lack of confidence in their competence also causes them to be vulnerable to criticism from important members of their social network and to sanctions against breastfeeding in our culture.[31]

The women who seem to respond best to education about the benefits of breastfeeding are those who are already determined to breastfeed, those who feel self-confident and efficacious. Information about the myriad advantages of breastfeeding will further strengthen the conviction of these women to breastfeed. Education alone is less likely to influence those women preoccupied with doubts about their competency as mothers.

Bandura states that individuals draw on several types of information in building their perception of self-efficacy. Two of these are past performance accomplishments and vicarious experience.[32] Women who have no previous parenting experience and have grown up in families where breastfeeding is not practiced have no past breastfeeding performance accomplishments and no vicarious experience of breastfeeding. Therefore, they are less likely to perceive themselves as competent breastfeeders even if their self-efficacy rating is generally high. They are breaking new ground.

Past performance accomplishments cannot be altered. However, there are ways for women to gain vicarious experience with breastfeeding. Breastfeeding can be made visible through use of posters and videos in hallways and in waiting, counseling, and examination rooms. Images should include women of all races and ethnicities. Breastfeeding women can be welcomed to nurse in public places. Images of and information about breastfeeding can be included in elementary and secondary school health education curricula. Media sources can be encouraged to incorporate positive depictions of breastfeeding women.

Breastfeeding Peer Counseling: Integrating Education and Social Learning

Breastfeeding peer counseling programs provide a powerful forum for education within relationships. The history of breastfeeding peer counseling in the United States began with the formation of La Leche League in 1956. La Leche League is grounded in the concept of mother-to-mother support. Leaders are mothers who have been trained by other leaders. A special feature of leader training is the process of active listening, a technique which brings the mothers' experience into the forefront. La Leche League is credited with beginning the renaissance of breastfeeding in the United States. The work of groups like La Leche League have helped to create space, similar to the original breastfeeding-friendly extended family, which gives support and strength to those choosing breastfeeding.

La Leche League groups are well distributed in suburban, middle-class neighborhoods. Many activists for breastfeeding in low-income and urban communities strive to replicate this model in their communities. Breastfeeding support groups and peer counselor programs have since become popular in WIC Programs, other Maternal-Child Health Programs, and hospitals.

Social Learning Aspects of Peer Learning Programs

Support groups and peer counseling programs provide women with many learning tools. One tool is vicarious experience. Peer counselor programs train and employ experienced women who have successfully breastfed a child or children to counsel and support other women. Counselors are trained not just in the basics of breastfeeding, but most importantly in counseling and communication skills. Peer counselors often model breastfeeding and mothering behaviors to pregnant women and new mothers by attending prenatal classes and clinics to nurse their babies in these settings and to share their experience. Reflecting on the confidence of these counselors can be personally empowering for many women.

Peer counseling programs provide the tool of connection with other women. The relational model of female development has identified that women experience emotional growth in connection with other women.[33] Many women benefit just from being in the presence of others who speak with a genuine voice. Women learn through listening to the way that others perceive their situation, the strategies that others develop to deal with problems and challenges, and the outcomes of these strategies. They learn that they are not alone, that other women share their fears and doubts as well as their hopes and aspirations.

Another aspect of the peer experience is known as *homophily.* Rogers affirms that people are most able to accept new ideas when they come from people who they perceive to be similar to themselves.[34] Describing peer counselors as indigenous health care workers (IHCW), Giblin writes:

> Indigenous qualities include, in most general terms, the possession of the social, environmental, and ethnic qualities of a subculture, and, in more specific terms, a sharing with a client of a verbal and non-verbal language, an understanding of a community's health beliefs and barriers to health care services, and an enhanced empathy with and responsibility toward a community and its health service needs. Indigenous qualities are thought to enhance an IHCW's role as a liaison between professional and lay health languages, attitudes, and behaviors, and the possession of an active and credible role in the life of the client.[35]

Information presented by someone perceived to be a peer may have more weight than that delivered by a person perceived to be different; e.g., an authority figure. Vicarious experience may resonate more when it is perceived to be genuine.

Bryant and colleagues write of the power of vicarious peer experience:

> In contrast to their responses when asked individually in a clinic situation, when most report that they intend to bottle-feed, women in group situations are less decisive and express interest in knowing more about breastfeeding. In many groups, women who initially indicated a preference for bottle-feeding changed their decision after listening to other participants speak convincingly of breastfeeding's advantages. In making their decisions, women weigh breastfeeding's advantages with a variety of barriers that they must overcome to lactate successfully.[36]

To address the tremendous racial, ethnic, and economic disparities in current breastfeeding rates, peer counselors and leaders from a wide range of racial, ethnic, and economic backgrounds are needed in order to provide vicarious, peer role models for all women. Peer counseling programs also provide a natural training ground for future professionals and paraprofessionals.

Impact of Breastfeeding Peer Counseling Programs

The impact of breastfeeding peer counselor programs has yet to be extensively studied. However, several articles have been published reviewing the local impact of such programs. Long and colleagues studied the impact of a peer counselor program in a Utah Native American

WIC participant population. Women who participated in the experimental group were more likely to initiate breastfeeding (84 percent experimental versus 70 percent of controls) and to be breastfeeding at three months postpartum (49 percent versus 36 percent).[37] Long and colleagues write: "Peer counselors may be especially important in the Native American population, where women in their traditional culture learned from or were taught by their mothers and doulas. Peer counselors may be even more beneficial to urban Native Americans, who are more likely to lack family support than are those living on rural reservations."[38]

Gross and colleagues examined the impact of peer counseling and motivational videotapes on duration of breastfeeding in an African American WIC population.[39] They found that women in all experimental groups were more likely to continue breastfeeding at 8 and 16 weeks postpartum than those who were in the control group.

Arlotti and colleagues measured the impact of peer support on duration and exclusivity of breastfeeding and found rates of both to be greater in women who received peer support.[40] Both initiation and duration have been shown to be enhanced by peer counseling programs by other researchers.[41]

Improving the visibility of breastfeeding and enhancing the development of self-efficacy and connection among women are tremendously valuable strategies for helping individuals to reclaim breastfeeding. These strategies in themselves cannot change many other hurdles standing in the path of childbearing women: short maternity leaves, lack of protection of rights of working, breastfeeding women, shunning of women breastfeeding in public, and others. Much work needs to be done in reweaving breastfeeding into the fiber of this nation—improving laws, revitalizing social support, and more. Implementation of strategies such as peer counseling programs cannot remove all of the barriers to breastfeeding. However, the experience of being involved with a grass roots support program such as breastfeeding peer counseling can serve as a laboratory for social change. Incremental social change occurs when each individual woman is well supported in her choice to breastfeed.

On Cape Cod in Massachusetts, a group of newly trained peer counselors expanded their volunteer activities beyond hours of weekly consultations to develop a breastfeeding corner at a local county fair. The success of this endeavor led the group to initiate a regional evaluation of the breastfeeding-friendliness restaurants and shopping centers. This then led them to propose sponsorship of statewide legislation regarding women's rights to breastfeed in public. There seems to be no end to the power of women who have discovered their self-efficacy, and the power of connection. Empowered women can change the world.

Individual Counseling Strategies

Cultural competency is an important strategy for overcoming disparities of all types. Cultural competency describes "the interpersonal skills and attitudes that enable individuals to increase their understanding and appreciation of the rich and fluid nature of culture and of differences and similarities within, among, and between cultures and individuals . . . [Cultural competency] is a process that . . . providers must learn to adapt to each new individual encounter."[42]

Cultural competency is another form of literacy that caregivers need to develop and expand continuously. Each new client one encounters can be seen as a new story to be revealed.

The first step toward developing cultural competency occurs when the caregiver undertakes self-assessment, seeking to identify and remain conscious of his or her own cultural values and biases.[43]

Exploring the client's viewpoint is key in arriving at mutually acceptable understanding of the situations and problems and in the development of appropriate care plans. Several sources have identified general medical beliefs and values of different cultures.[44] Such information can provide a framework for initial exploration with clients. However, while it is possible to generalize about the experience of groups of people, it is impossible to predict the meaning of an experience for any individual. Truly culturally competent caregivers make no assumptions about the experience, practices, or viewpoints of others, but ask each client they encounter to help them understand the situation and possible solutions through the client's eyes.

Levin and colleagues cite an acronym, ETHNIC, used to denote a framework for components of culturally competent care.[45] The ETHNIC framework for breastfeeding caregivers is paraphrased in Figure 9.3.

Additional Strategies

Additional strategies for communication are summarized below:

- Strive to establish an environment of trust and respect with all clients, asking questions rather than making assumptions and being sensitive to differing customs regarding body language, eye contact, touching, etc. Modifying one's own communication strategies can help build a relationship with the client. When we reach out to women by attempting to speak their language (both figuratively and literally), women are more likely to share their inner thoughts and realities with us.[46]
- Talk with all women about breastfeeding. Avoid making assumptions of whether or not they will be receptive to information about breastfeeding. It is also very important to talk about breastfeeding

Explanation:	Ask: "What do you think may have caused this problem/ situation? What do your family and friends say about it? What concerns you most about this problem/situation?"
Treatments:	Ask: "What kinds of treatments have you tried for this problem/situation? Would you tell me about any special things that you do (or avoid doing) to solve this problem? What kind of treatment do you think you need from me?"
Healers:	Ask: "Who else might help you with this problem/ situation?" (Probe for alternative or folk healers, family, or friends.)
Negotiate:	Try to find options that will be mutually acceptable that incorporate the beneficial familial beliefs, rather than contradicting them.
Intervention:	Together with the woman, develop an intervention strategy that will solve the problem.
Collaboration:	Collaborate with the woman, her family, other care givers, and community resources.

FIGURE 9.3   ETHNIC: A Mnemonic Device for Culturally Competent Care. *Source:* Adapted from Levin, S. J. et al. 2000. Appendix A: Useful Clinical Interviewing Mnemonics. Patient Care Special Issue, "Caring for Diverse Population: Breaking Down Barriers," May 15, 2000: 189.

with women who report they have breastfed a previous child rather than assuming it was a good experience for them. Biancuzzo writes, "It's important to learn how long she breastfed, and whether she found it a satisfactory or unsatisfactory experience."[47]

- Invite dialogue with the client.[48] One author suggests saying, "If I tell you something and your mother has told you something different, please let me know and we'll see how we can work together."[49]
- Include partners and family members in encounters as much as possible.
- Establish communication plans. Identify when, where, and how follow-up will happen. If telephone communication is planned, specify who will call whom. Backup communication plans are helpful, as many women move frequently.
- Know that women experiencing stress may require additional counseling. Haider writes that "support is essential for all lactating mothers, women with familial or financial problems require special attention and extra counselling sessions so that they can be helped to identify how to achieve and sustain exclusive breast-feeding."[50] The interface with a breastfeeding caregiver may provide the only

link to other needed medical, nutritional, and/or social services and resources.

- Integrate breastfeeding follow-up with other services (e.g., pediatric follow-up) to the extent possible. Several researchers have shown that providing continuous lactation care within the framework of comprehensive prenatal, postpartum, and pediatric care is most effective in increasing incidence duration and exclusivity of breastfeeding.[51]
- Develop peer counseling programs, and refer women to them routinely. Peer counseling programs have been identified among the most effective strategies for breastfeeding promotion and preservation.

Health Systems Strategies

- Encourage training in breastfeeding and cultural competency for all health providers.
- Increase awareness of community breastfeeding support systems and services among health care providers.
- Address language and literacy barriers by providing multilingual staff, interpretive services, and translated educational materials. Display posters and pictures of women of all races and ethnicities served.
- Identify individuals within underserved communities who are willing to serve as "cultural brokers," providing cultural interpretation when needed.[52]
- Broaden knowledge about the reality of clients' lives. Summarizing findings of focus group research, Underwood and colleagues write "it was apparent that professionals and staff involved in this project needed to gain an understanding of common infant feeding practices of low-income African American women; a greater awareness of the values, beliefs, and health care practices of the population; and a greater understanding of the impact of poverty on the families within the targeted community."[53]
- Encourage cultural assessment of underserved communities to identify the major values, health beliefs, and practices of target populations.[54] Cultural assessment should include examination of communication strategies (verbal and nonverbal), space (comfortable physical distance between speakers), social organization (the important groupings in an individual's life), and time (orientation to the future).
- Encourage systems and providers to study the impact of health care practices (e.g., hospital practices, distribution of discharge bags and formula samples) on breastfeeding outcomes.

- Explore barriers to breastfeeding through ongoing dialogue with community members, and use this information to design and refine programs and strategies, targeting identified barriers, concerns, and needs. Writing of their experience in understanding why Hawaiian women weaned early, Novotny and colleagues state, "We can identify a time-associated phenomenon whereby formula introduction increased the risk of breastfeeding cessation. . . . In Hawaii, programs that address how and when to introduce foods, use of formula, and management of outside employment and breastfeeding should be made available to those groups of women at risk for early weaning to lengthen their duration of breastfeeding."[55] In a different study, Kistin and colleagues found "that the content of successful breast-feeding [education] among black urban poor women should stress the following: that breast-feeding is healthiest for newborns; that a woman can have a busy life and still breast-feed; and that there is much misinformation about diet, smoking, and contraindications to breast-feeding that needs to be cleared up so women can make informed choices about feeding their infants."[56]

Summary

Dr. Wanda Jones, Deputy Assistant Secretary for Health and Director of the Office on Women's Health, summarized the strategies needed to overcome disparities and build an environment of universal support for breastfeeding:

> The Healthy People objectives will be realized only when we work together to put in place culturally appropriate strategies to promote breastfeeding, with particular emphasis on education and support from health care professionals, employers and family members, especially fathers and grandmothers.[57]

Work must be done in rebuilding a society where breastfeeding is the cultural norms, but the rewards of this work will be far reaching in improving the health of our nation.

References and Notes

1. United States Department of Health and Human Services. 2000. *Healthy People 2010: Understanding and Improving Health*. Washington, DC: Author, Government Printing Office.
2. Office of the United States Surgeon General. October 30, 2000. News Release. Washington, DC: Office on Women's Health.

3. United States Department of Health and Human Services. 2000. *Healthy People 2010: Conference Edition—Volumes I and II.* Washington, DC, Author.

4. Office of the United States Surgeon General, 2000.

5. Forste, R. et al. 2001. The decision to breastfeed in the United States: Does race matter? *Peds.* 108: 291.

6. Ryan, A. S. 1997. The Resurgence of Breastfeeding in the United States. *Peds.* 99(4): e12.

7. Baydar, N. et al. 1997. WIC Infant Feeding Practices Study: Summary of Findings. Alexandria, VA: United States Department of Agriculture.

8. Ryan, A. S. 1997.

9. Romero-Gwynn, E. 1989. Breast-feeding patterns among Indochinese immigrants in Northern California. *Am. J. Dis. Child.* 243: 804.

10. Ibid.

11. Kocturk, T., and R. Zetterstrom. 1986. Breastfeeding among Turkish mothers living in suburbs of Istanbul and Stockholm: A comparison. *Acta. Paediat. Scand.* 75: 216.

12. Romero-Gwynn, E. 1989.

13. Romero-Gwynn, E., and L. Carias. 1989. Breast-feeding intentions and practices among Hispanic mothers in Southern California. *Peds.* 84: 626. Balcazar, H. et al. 1995. What predicts breastfeeding intention in Mexican-American and Non-Hispanic white women? Evidence from a national survey. *Birth* 22(2): 74.

14. Raissin, D. K. et al. 1993. Acculturation and breastfeeding on the United States-Mexico border. *Am. J. Med. Sci.* 306(1): 28.

15. Gunnlaugsson, G., and J. Einarsdottir. 1993. Colostrum and ideas about bad milk: A case study from Guinea-Bissau. *Soc. Sci. Med.* 326(3): 283.

16. Tuttle, C. R., and K. G. Dewey.1994. Determinants of infant feeding choices among Southeast Asian immigrants in northern California. *J. Am. Diet. Assoc.* 94:282.

17. Carter, P. 1995. *Feminism, Breasts and Breast-feeding.* New York: St. Martin's Press.

18. Bernstein, N. 1999. Trial begins for mother in breast-fed infant's starvation death. *New York Times,* April 28, 1999.

19. Helliker, K. 1994. Dying for milk: Some mothers, trying in vain to breast-feed starve their infants. "Yuppie Syndrome" among well-meaning parents stems from bad advice: A generation of perfectionists. *Wall Street Journal,* July 22, 1994: 1.

20. Gorman, C. When breast-feeding fails: Low-milk syndrome poses a rare but frightening risk. *Time,* August 22, 1994: 63.

21. Bernstein, N. 1999. Placing the blame in an infant's death: mother faces trial after baby dies from lack of breast milk. *New York Times.* March 15, 1999: B1.

22. Bernstein, N. 1999. Bronx woman convicted in starving of her breast-fed son. *New York Times.* May 20, 1999: B1.

23. Kogan, M. D. et al. 1994. Racial disparities in reported prenatal care advice from health care providers. *Am. J. Pub. Health* 84: 82.

24. Armotrading, D. C. et al. 1992. Impact of WIC utilization rate on breast-feeding among international students at a large university. *J. Am. Diet. Assoc.* 92(3): 352.

25. Shand, N., and Y. Kosawa. 1984. Breast-feeding as cultural or personal decision: Sources of information and actual success in Japan and the United States. *J. Biosoc. Sci.* 15: 654.

26. Kistin, N. et al. 1990. Breast-feeding rates among black urban low-income women: Effect of prenatal education. *Pediatrics* 86: 741.

27. The United States Department of Agriculture's Breastfed Babies Welcome Here, and Loving Support Campaigns are examples of programs that have targeted key strategic individuals who influence the feeding choices of pregnant and breastfeeding women: partners, family, friends, and day-care providers.

28. Lapinski, M. K., and K. Witte. 1998. Health communication campaigns. In L. D. Jackson and B. K. Duffy, eds. *Health Communication Research: A Guide to Developments and Directions.* Westport, CT: Greenwood Press.

29. Friedman, H. S. et al. 1990. In S. A. Shumaker, E. B. Schron, and J. K. Ockene, eds. *The Handbook of Health Behavior Change.* New York: Springer Publishing Company.

30. Bandura, A. 1989. Perceived self-efficacy in the exercise of control over AIDS infection. In V. M. Mays, G. W. Albee, and S. S. Schneider, eds. *Primary Prevention of AIDS: Psychological Approaches.* Newbury Park, CA: Sage Publications.

31. Bryant, C. A. et al. 1992. A strategy for promoting breastfeeding among economically disadvantaged women and adolescents. *NAACOG's Clinical Issues in Perinatal and Women's Health Issues: Breastfeeding* 3(4): 723.

32. Bandura, A. 1977. Self-efficacy: Toward a unifying theory of behavioral change. *Psychological Review* 84: 191.

33. Jordan, J. V. et al. 1991. *Women's Growth in Connection: Writings from the Stone Center.* New York: The Guilford Press.

34. Rogers, D. M. 1995. *Diffusion of Innovations,* 4th edition. New York: Free Press.

35. Giblin, P. T. 1989. Effective utilization and evaluation of Indigenous Health Care Workers. *Pub. Hlth. Report* 104(4): 361.

36. Bryant, C. A. et al. 1992. 724.

37. Long, D. G. et al. 1995. Peer counselor program increases breastfeeding rates in Utah Native American WIC population. *J. Hum. Lact.* 11(4): 279.

38. Ibid.

39. Gross, S. M. et al. 1998. Counseling and motivational videotapes increase duration of breast-feeding in African-American WIC participants who initiate breast-feeding. *J. Am. Diet. Assoc.* 98: 143.

40. Arlotti, J. P. et al. 1998. Breastfeeding among low-income women with and without peer support. *J Comm Health Nurs* 15(3): 163.

41. Schafer, E. et al. 1998. Volunteer peer counselors increase breastfeeding duration among rural low-income women. *Birth* 25(2): 101.
Shaw, E., and J. Kaczorowski. 1991. The effect of a peer counseling program on breastfeeding initiation and longevity in a low-income rural population. *J. Hum. Lact.* 15(1): 19.

42. Chesapeake Institute. 1994. *National Agenda for Achieving Better Results for Children and Youth with Serious Emotional Disturbance.* URL: *http://cecp.air.org/resources/ntlagend.html.* Accessed 01/27/00.

43. Gabriel, A. et al. 1986. Cultural values and biomedical knowledge: Choices in infant feeding. *Soc. Sci. Med.* 23(5): 501.

44. Taylor, M. M. 1985. *Transcultural Aspects of Breastfeeding—USA.* Lactation Consultant Series, Unit 2. Wayne, NJ: Avery Publishing Group. Waxler-Morrison, N. et al. 1990. *Cross-Cultural Caring: A Handbook for Health Professionals.* Vancouver, BC: University of British Columbia. Winikoff, B. et al., eds. 1988. *Feeding Infants in Four Societies: Causes and Consequences of Mothers' Choices.* New York: Greenwood Press.

45. Levin, S. J. et al. 2000. Appendix A: Useful Clinical Interviewing Mnemonics. Patient Care Special Issue, "Caring for Diverse Populations: Breaking Down Barriers," May 15: 189.

46. Giger, J. N., and R. Davidhizar. 1990. Transcultural nursing assessment: A method for advancing nursing practice. *Int. Nurs. Rev.* 37: 199.

47. Biancuzzo, M. 2001. *Helping Mothers Choose and Initiate Breastfeeding.* Herndon, VA: WMC Worldwide, LLC.

48. Abramson, R. 1992. Cultural sensitivity in the promotion of breastfeeding. *NAACOG Clin. Issues* 3(4): 718.

49. Taylor, M. M. 1985. *Transcultural Aspects of Breastfeeding—USA.* Lactation Consultant Series, Unit 2. Wayne, NJ: Avery Publishing Group.

50. Haider, R. et al. 1997. Reasons for failure of breast-feeding counselling: Mothers' perspectives in Bangladesh. *Bull World Health Org.* 75(3): 191.

51. Balcazar, H. et al. 1995. What predicts breastfeeding intention in Mexican-American and non-Hispanic white women? Evidence from a national survey. *Birth* 22(2): 74–80.
    Kistin, N. et al. 1990. Breastfeeding rates among black urban low-income women: Effect of prenatal education. *Pediatrics* 86(5): 741.
    Brent, N. B. et al. 1995. Breastfeeding in a low-income population. *Arch. Pediatr. Adolesc. Med.* 149: 798.
    Lutter, C. K. et al. 1997. The effectiveness of a hospital-based program to promote exclusive breast-feeding among low-income women in Brazil. *Am. J. Public Health* 87: 659.

52. Fadiman, A. 1997. *The Spirit Catches You and You Fall Down: A Hmong Child, her American Doctors, and the Collision of Two Cultures.* New York: Noonday Press.

53. Underwood, S. et al. 1997. Infant feeding practices of low-income African American women in a central city community. *J. Comm. Health Nurs.* 14(3): 189.

54. Young, S. A., and M. Kaufman. 1988. Promoting breastfeeding at a migrant health center. *Am. J. Public Health* 78(5): 523.

55. Novotny, R. et al. 2000. Breastfeeding duration in a multiethnic population in Hawaii. Birth 27: 91.

56. Kistin, N. et al. 1990. Breast-feeding rates among black urban low-income: Effect of prenatal education. *Peds.* 86: 741.

57. Office of the United States Surgeon General. *News Release.* October 30, 2000. Washington, DC: Office on Women's Health.

CHAPTER TEN

LACTACTION AND THE WORKPLACE

Zoë Maja McInerney, M.A., C.L.C.

This chapter explores the relationship between maternal employment and breastfeeding. It includes a brief review of women's participation in the workforce as well as research on the relationship between employment and breastfeeding initiation and duration. Finally, it explores government regulations and employer accommodations that are intended to support breastfeeding women in the workplace.

This text has covered in depth the physiological and emotional benefits of breastfeeding. This chapter takes the position that breastfeeding is best and should be supported and encouraged. Mothers of young children make up a greater proportion of the workforce than ever before, so the question of how to combine breastfeeding and employment is growing more relevant. Research has shown that mothers who return to work and are not able to continue breastfeeding as long as they had planned report significantly more feelings of sadness or depression and guilt.[1] Employers also have financial benefits when their employees breastfeed their children. It is, therefore, in everyone's best interest to support women who wish to continue breastfeeding on their return to paid employment.

Women's Workforce Participation

The composition of the United States workforce has radically changed over the course of the past century. The workforce now includes more women than ever before. In 1950, women comprised only 30 percent of the civilian workforce. By 1980 that number had risen to 43 percent, and in 2025 the proportion of women in the workforce is projected to reach 48 percent.[2] From 1978 to 1998 the number of married mothers of young children working full time outside the home increased from 14 percent to 35 percent.[3] In 1997, 58 percent of mothers with children were working or looking for work.[4] Women are projected to increase their membership in the labor force at a faster rate than men from 46 percent in 1997 to 47 percent in 2006.[5]

The number of married women with children entering into paid labor has increased more dramatically in the 1990s than the number of single women entering the workforce.[6] Mothers of young children are now more likely to work than at any other time in the past.[7] Unsurprisingly, most women report that they work primarily because their family needs the money.[8] Many dual-income families could not support themselves if forced to rely on a single income, and single parents have no other income on which to rely. Whatever the causes, the changes are a reality and the increase in the number of working mothers affects how and if women breastfeed their babies.

Relationship Between Breastfeeding and Mothers' Employment

Considerable disagreement is apparent in the literature about how returning to work affects duration of breastfeeding. We know that maternal employment is increasingly common and likely to increase more. Some researchers have made the assumption that breastfeeding and work are incompatible, but on closer inspection of the literature, some have found employment status to be unrelated to age of weaning. Many women may not be aware that resources are available to help women who choose to breastfeed and work.

Maternal employment is reported in some studies to have a negative effect on breastfeeding duration. Ryan and Martinez, of Ross Laboratories, conducted a large national survey of working mothers.[9] Looking only at mothers employed full time and those not employed outside the home, they found that at six months of age, only 10 percent of the infants of employed mothers were still being breastfed compared to 24 percent of nonworking mothers. However, as the researchers point out, they did not define the term "full time" so they do not know how many hours the employed mothers worked nor whether they were separated from their babies during their work day. They also did not collect data on how soon they returned to work after giving birth, a factor that other studies have shown to be relevant.

A large telephone survey of new mothers conducted through John Hopkins University found significant differences between employed and nonemployed women. They found that at six to twelve weeks post-partum, 48 percent of employed mothers who had initiated breastfeeding were still breastfeeding, compared to 68 percent of nonemployed mothers. They also found that the number of hours worked had an effect on duration. Mothers working twenty or fewer hours were significantly more likely to still be breastfeeding at six to twelve weeks postpartum than mothers who worked more than twenty hours. Unfortunately, how supportive the participants rated their workplace made no difference in the continuation of breastfeeding.[10]

Another study, which found a negative effect of maternal employment on breastfeeding, examined resident physicians. Miller and colleagues[11] realized that 23 percent of women residents had a first child during their residency and examined the effect of residency on their breastfeeding practices and experiences. They found that while an unusually high number initiated breastfeeding (80 percent, compared to the national average of 60 percent), that number dropped to 40 percent after two months and 15 percent at six months. By far the most common reason cited for weaning was "schedule did not permit." While this study is interesting for physician and resident populations, the results may not be relevant to working mothers in general. The long hours of a resident physician are unlike most other professions, and the women in this study were often required to be away from their infants for twenty-five or more hours at a time. The schedule constraints on these women may be extreme compared to those of other working women and make it difficult to continue breastfeeding their children. Most working mothers are required to spend far fewer hours away from their children, making breastfeeding a much more viable option.

Contrary to the studies mentioned above, all research does not show returning to employment to have a negative effect on duration of breastfeeding. Several studies have found higher rates of breastfeeding among mothers who worked outside the home compared to mothers who stayed at home. One study found that women who were working at the time of the study had breastfed longer than those who did not work outside the home at the time of the study.[12] However, since this survey was administered after weaning and it provides no information about the timing of their return to work, it cannot tell us how work itself affected breastfeeding. It does provide an indication that planning to return to work was not an inhibiting factor in the duration of breastfeeding.

Another study found planned employment to have no effect on the plan to breastfeed. The researchers surveyed newly delivered mothers about their plans regarding infant feeding, planned duration of breastfeeding, anticipated factors which might affect the duration of breastfeeding, the father's attitude regarding breastfeeding, and infant feeding choices of close friends and family members. Intentions regarding returning to work were not related to the participants' decisions to breastfeed. The only factor that was significantly related to feeding choice was the fathers' attitude toward breastfeeding. Seventy-five percent of babies born to fathers who totally approved of breastfeeding were breastfed compared to only 8 percent of babies whose fathers were indifferent or disapproving. Unfortunately, this study did not look at the behavior of participants, only intentions. Therefore, we cannot conclude from the results that working has no effect on breastfeeding, only that the intention to work has no relationship to the intention to breastfeed.[13]

Hight-Laukaran and colleagues examined the hypothesis that it may not be work itself that affects mothers' ability to breastfeed, but particular attributes of work that make breastfeeding more difficult.[14] Specifically, they examined not only employment status; they also asked women whether they were able to take their baby to work with them. They surveyed women from 15 developing nations in Africa, Asia, the Near East, Latin America, and the Caribbean. Using epidemiological methodology they determined the amount of risk of using breast milk substitutes attributable to employment that always separated the mother from her baby. They found that the percentage of this risk attributable to employment ranged from 0.74 percent in the Dominican Republic to 20.9 percent in Namibia. In 10 of the 15 countries, less than 5 percent of the risk of using breast milk substitutes was attributable to the mothers' employment. This indicates that employment may not be as much of a factor in the duration of breastfeeding as many believe.

These researchers are not the only ones to wonder if the attributes of work, rather than work itself, have an affect on breastfeeding choice and duration. One of these attributes, specifically the number of hours worked per week, was investigated by Fein and Roe.[15] They found that mothers who were working full time at three months postpartum had significantly lower amounts of both initiation rates and duration of breastfeeding than mothers who were not working at that time. However, the breastfeeding initiation and duration of mothers who worked part time was not different from nonemployed mothers. The investigators concluded that working part-time was an effective strategy for mothers who returned to work and wanted to continue breastfeeding.

Auerbach and Guss[16] found that timing of mothers' return to work had more of an effect on breastfeeding than the number of hours worked. Mothers in the study who returned to work earlier than sixteen weeks postpartum were more likely to wean early than mothers who had longer maternity leaves. They also found that mothers who worked part time were more likely to nurse their babies for more than a year compared to mothers who were employed full time. A comparison of the two showed the timing of return to have a stronger effect on breastfeeding duration. Mothers who worked full time, but not until after sixteen weeks, breastfed longer than mothers who worked part time but returned to work earlier.

The finding of the previous study is supported by another study that found the duration of maternity leave to be positively associated with the duration of breastfeeding. This national survey also looked at the effects of maternal employment on breastfeeding initiation and duration. These researchers found that women employed before delivery were more likely to initiate breastfeeding than those not previously employed. Returning to work within a year postpartum had no effect on breastfeeding initiation rates. However, mothers who returned to work before six weeks postpartum were less likely to breastfeed. They also found that duration of maternity leave was strongly associated with duration of breastfeeding and also that Caucasian professional women were the most likely to nurse their child for a longer period of time. The study's authors speculate that this may be because professional women might have greater control over their work environment and more flexibility in combining work and family demands.[17]

There is no definitive answer to the question of how to combine maternal employment and breastfeeding. The research has produced conflicting conclusions. There are studies that seem to show a negative effect of work on breastfeeding initiation and duration. However, other research has indicated that there is little or no relationship between mothers' employment status and breastfeeding success. Other research indicates that mothers who work may be more likely to breastfeed. So far, there is no absolute right answer. However, given the absence of any proof that women who work are not able to successfully breastfeed, we should stop assuming that the two activities are mutually exclusive. Instead of deciding that women who return to work while still nursing infants must stop breastfeeding, there should be an effort to support these women, to make it easier to continue breastfeeding for as long as they choose. The studies discussed above have indicated that the timing of a woman's return to work may have an effect on her ability to continue breastfeeding, as can the number of hours worked after her return. Also, the assumption is generally made that employment means total separation from the child. This does not have to be true. Through minor accommodations, often breastfeeding and employment can be combined successfully.

Promoting Breastfeeding for Employed Mothers

Often what determines the timing of a mother's return to work after the birth of a child is the length of her maternity leave. Evidence suggests that if mothers can stay at home for at least four months they will have a greater chance of successfully continuing to breastfeed.[18] One explanation for this is that sixteen weeks is generally long enough to establish a good milk supply. Also, the mother has probably solved several temporary breastfeeding crises already and has the confidence to survive any others that may occur.

Unfortunately, women are not always guaranteed maternity leave. Many countries have laws about the time women may take away from work and still be assured of returning to their same jobs. In the United States, maternity leave is legislated under the Family and Medical Leave Act. Enacted in 1993, the act mandates the right to twelve weeks of unpaid leave and job reinstatement upon return for both men and women. Leave can be taken for a variety of family and medical reasons, including the birth or adoption of a child, acquisition of a foster child, a serious illness, or to care for a child, spouse, or parent with a serious illness.[19] However, because of restrictions on eligibility, many women are not covered under the Family and Medical Leave Act and thus are not entitled to any maternity leave. Women working for businesses with fewer than 50 employees, those working part time (defined as fewer than 24 hours a week), and anyone working for their employer for less than a year are not covered. It is estimated that under the current restrictions, only about half of working women in the United States are eligible for maternity leave. Many women who may qualify for the twelve weeks of unpaid leave are unable to take it for financial reasons. Unpaid leave is only useful in families who have another income that is able to support them during the leave time. Families of this sort have become rare, and low-income families often rely heavily, if not solely, on the mother's income. In states where partial wage replacement was available through temporary disability insurance, low-income women were more likely to take longer maternity leaves.[20]

International maternity leave support is stronger. The International Labor Organization (ILO) exists to promote social justice and labor rights. It regulates labor issues by deciding on standards contained in conventions which, if ratified by member nations, are binding. In 1919, when the organization was first established, the ILO recognized the needs of childbearing women and called for twelve weeks of paid maternity leave, free medical care during pregnancy, right of return after leave, and nursing breaks during the workday in its Maternity Protection Convention. This original convention provided for women employed in commerce and industry. In 1921 the ILO expanded these rights to agricultural workers, and in the 1950s the provisions were strengthened and expanded to women who worked at home and those who worked on plantations.[21]

Individual countries vary in the amount of maternity leave and in how it is distributed. Scandinavian countries provide leave to either parent. In Sweden eighteen months of leave is available to be shared by both parents. Whichever parent is taking leave can receive 90 percent of their salary for fifteen months.[22]

Israel has a long tradition of support for employed mothers. In 1954 the Women's Work Law mandated a full twelve weeks of paid maternity leave, at least six weeks of which must be taken after childbirth. The birth of twins adds two weeks to the maternity leave, and employers are prohibited from firing pregnant women before they take their leave. Either parent has the option to take an unpaid leave of absence for up to twelve months, after which they must be allowed to return to their jobs with no penalty.[23]

In the United Kingdom prior to 1976, women were generally expected to leave the workforce after having children. However, the Employment Protection Acts of 1976 and 1978 introduced legally sanctioned maternity leave. Under these acts, women who have worked for the same employer for two years have the right to six weeks of maternity leave paid at 90 percent of their regular wages. They also have the option of an additional twelve weeks for a small flat-rate payment and an additional unpaid 22 weeks. The British system has limitations similar to those of the U.S. system. The length of service requirement disqualifies many women, and fears of a negative impact on business led to an exemption for smaller companies in spite of the fact that most employers report no difficulties caused by providing maternity leave. Another criticism of the British system has to do with the lack of flexibility in the number of hours worked upon return.[24]

Other nations have policies that allow some maternity leave to be taken as part-time work, easing the transition from home to work for both mother and baby. This kind of policy is particularly beneficial to breastfeeding mothers. The research discussed earlier in this chapter indicates that the time of return to work and the number of hours worked when mothers first return can affect the duration of breastfeeding. Providing paid maternity leave makes it possible for mothers to take the leave they are entitled to take. Allowing some leave to be taken as reduced work hours upon the return to work may make it easier for some mothers to continue breastfeeding.

Another way to support breastfeeding mothers who return to work is to minimize the separation from the baby. This can be done through several different workplace accommodations, including on-site child care, allowing women to return to work part time, work at home or telecommute, providing facilities for women to keep their babies with them in the workplace (sometimes referred to as a creche), and providing a place to pump and store breast milk. Research done on a strategy for continuing to breastfeed while working referred to it as juggling.[25] Juggling mothers manage to breastfeed their babies and work concurrently, as opposed to a "serial strategy" in which mothers breastfeed, wean, then return to work. Strategies for successful juggling include mothers working at home with the baby, the baby going to work with the mother, the mother going to the baby during the work day, or the baby being brought to the mother during the work day. Another option is pumping breast milk during the work day for a baby who is being cared for elsewhere. Mothers can help maintain their milk supply for infants being fed elsewhere by pumping milk. However, this approach has been popular almost exclusively in the U.S., where options such as nursing breaks and bringing babies to work are rarely discussed. While pumping milk for babies meets infants' nutritional needs, the emotional benefits for both mother and child are ignored by these solutions.[26]

In the research on juggling, mothers who were able to combine breastfeeding and work or pump at work and save the milk (to be fed to the baby later) breastfed longer than women who did not use either of these strategies. Women using these juggling strategies were also nursing more frequently each day than women who did not pump or breastfeed at work. Women who employed these strategies tended to be older and more educated. They were less embarrassed about breastfeeding and less likely to have had early breastfeeding problems. Women who juggled for longer periods of time were more likely to have the baby with them while working. Juggling enabled mothers to breastfeed longer, which is in the best interest of the mother and child. Women were able to juggle more easily if they worked part time, if they were able to breastfeed during the work day, and if they were able to pump and save the milk.[27]

If we intend to support breastfeeding mothers in the workplace, providing a place to pump and an adequate storage place is only part of the solution. Unfortunately, even this small workplace accommodation is rare, and it is usually the only option that is considered. It will not be feasible for every working woman to have her baby with her at the workplace, but there ought to be more discussion about when and where it is a possibility.

A bill has recently been passed by the U.S. Congress that gives women the right to breastfeed in some public places. Championed by Rep. Carolyn Maloney (D-NY), the bill guarantees women the right to nurse on any federal property on which they are permitted. This legislation was enacted in response to nursing mothers being asked to leave national parks and similar public places. Unfortunately, this bill has nothing to say about private property or the workplace.

Two bills currently being reviewed in committee do relate to breast-feeding in the workplace. The first, Breastfeeding Promotion and Employers' Tax Incentive Act of 1999, seeks to give employers incentives to encourage breastfeeding by providing a safe and private environment for women to nurse or pump breastmilk. The second, Pregnancy Discrimination Act Amendment of 1999, tries to protect breastfeeding under civil rights law, requiring that women cannot be fired or discriminated against in the workplace for expressing breast milk (or directly breastfeeding) during their own lunch or break time. If passed, these bills would provide legal support for women choosing to continue breastfeeding after returning to work.

Employer Benefits to Accommodating Breastfeeding

To those who well understand the benefits of breastfeeding, the encouragement of its continuation in working mothers is practical. Breastfeeding has numerous health-related and emotional benefits to both mother and child that should be supported and valued by our society. However, in an economy characterized by low unemployment and a shortage of highly skilled workers, women and men are encouraged to work more, and many employers may see maternity benefits as encouraging women to spend less time in the office. Some people may believe that breastfeeding and employment are incompatible. However, some accommodation in support of women choosing to breastfeed may have benefits that are overlooked by employers. Providing support and encouragement to breastfeeding women may mitigate problems such as turnover, absenteeism, and high health care costs.

Employee turnover is a costly problem for organizations. Not only can an experienced employee be lost in favor of an inexperienced one, but the costs of hiring and training a new employee can be prohibitive. Evidence exists that employees experiencing a conflict between work and family are more likely to leave their jobs.[28] Employees who perceive that their employers are supportive of their work and family difficulties are more likely to plan a return from maternity leave earlier and are generally more committed to their employer.[29] Although there is little research on the subject, perhaps breastfeeding women anticipating a supportive work environment may also be more likely to return following maternity leave. Maternity leave and support of breastfeeding is just one way to attract and retain employees.

Absenteeism is a problem incurring significant financial costs for employers.[30] Mothers who breastfeed their children tend to miss work because of an ill child less often than mothers who do not breastfeed.[31] Cohen and colleagues looked directly at the absence rates for breast-feeding and formula feeding employed mothers.[32] They found that breastfeeding mothers had fewer absences and that their infants had fewer and less severe illnesses. Formula feeding mothers had three times the number of single-day absences than breastfeeding mothers. This indicates a direct financial benefit for employers who support breastfeeding.

Breastfed children are sick less often than children fed with artificial baby milk[33] and the costs of child health care are higher for non-breastfed children.[34] These costs are then passed on to any employer who pays for the health insurance of employees' dependents. Providing support for employees who are breastfeeding their children saves money on health care costs.

Encouraging breastfeeding is in the best interest of the mother, baby, employer, and society. If companies were to make simple accommodations to make it easier for employees to breastfeed, they might see improvements in the absence and turnover rates of employees and in health care costs. These accommodations could be as small as providing a space for women to nurse or pump and store milk. They could be as extensive as paid maternity leaves, options to return to work part time, on-site child care, or arrangements for working at home. Whatever the accommodation, employers who support breastfeeding mothers will see benefits to their company, and the mothers and infants will benefit directly.

References

1. Chezem, J. et al. 1997. Maternal feelings after cessation of breastfeeding: Influence of factors related to employment and duration. *Journal of Perinatal and Neonatal Nursing,* 11(2): 61.
2. Fullerton, H. N. 1999. Labor force participation: 75 years of change, 1950–98 and 1998–2025. *Monthly Labor Review,* December:3.
3. Cohen, P. N., and S. M. Bianchi. 1999. Marriage, children, and women's employment: What do we know? *Monthly Labor Review,* December:22.
4. Bureau of Labor Statistics. 1998. Employment Characteristics of Families Summary. Current Population, Survey—Labor Force Statistics. Available: *http://stats.bls.gov/news.release/famee.nws.htm,* March:26.
5. Fullerton, H. N. 1999.
6. Hayghe, H. V. 1997. Developments in women's labor force participation. *Monthly Labor Review,* September:41.
7. Goodman, W. 1995. Boom in daycare industry the result of many social changes. *Monthly Labor Review,* August:3.

8. United States Department of Labor. 1994. *1993 Handbook on Women Workers: Trends and Issues*. Washington DC: United States Government Printing Office.

9. Ryan, A. S., and G. A. Martinez. 1989. Breast-Feeding and the working mother: A profile. *Pediatrics*, 83(4): 524.

10. Gielen, A. C. et al. 1991. Maternal employment during the early postpartum period: Effects on initiation and continuation of breast-feeding. *Pediatrics*, 87(3): 298.

11. Miller, N. H. et al. 1996. Breastfeeding practices among resident physicians. *Pediatrics*, 98 (3): 434.

12. Ståhlberg, M. R. 1985. Breast-feeding and social factors. *Acta. Pœdiatr. Scand.*, 74: 36.

13. Littman, H. et al. 1994. The decision to breastfeed: The importance of fathers' approval. *Clinical Pediatrics*, April: 214.

14. Hight-Laukaran, V. et al. 1996. The use of breast milk substitutes in developing countries: The impact of women's employment. *American Journal of Public Health*, 86(9): 1235.

15. Fein, S. B., and B. Roe. 1998. The effect of work status on initiation and duration of breast-feeding. *American Journal of Public Health*, 88(7): 1042.

16. Auerbach, K. G., and E. Guss. 1984. Maternal employment and breastfeeding: A study of 567 women's experiences. *American Journal of Diseases of Childhood*, 138: 958.

17. Visness, C. M., and K. I. Kennedy. 1997. Maternal employment and breast-feeding: Findings from the 1988 National Maternal and Infant Health Survey. *American Journal of Public Health*, 87(6): 945.

18. Auerbach, K. G., and E. Guss. 1984.

19. Galtry, J. 1997. Lactation and the labor market: Breastfeeding, labor market changes, and public policy in the United States. *Health Care for Women International*, 18: 467.
Smith, K. E., and A. Bachu. 1999. Women's Labor Force Attachment Patterns and Maternity Leave: A Review of the Literature. Population Division Working Paper No. 32. United States Bureau of the Census: Washington, DC.

20. Bond, J. T. et al. 1991. *Beyond the Parental Leave Debate, The Impact of Laws in Four States*. New York: The Families and Work Institute.

21. von Esterik, P., and L. Menon. 1996. *Being Mother Friendly: A Practical Guide for Working Women and Breastfeeding*. Penang, Malaysia: World Alliance for Breastfeeding Action.

22. Ibid.

23. Richter, J. 1992. Balancing work and family in Israel. In S. Zedick, ed., *Work, Families and Organizations*. San Francisco: Jossey-Bass. 362.

24. Lewis, S. 1992. Work and Families in the United Kingdom. In S. Zedick (Ed.) *Work, Families and Organizations*. San Francisco: Jossey-Bass. pp. 395.

25. Fein, S. B. 2001. Success of strategies to combine breastfeeding and employment. In *Giving Families Choices: Enacting Paid Family Leave*. Seminar at the Institute for Women's Policy Research, Washington, DC.

26. Galtry, J. 1997.
27. Fein, S. B. 2001.
    Bar-Yam, N. B. 1998. Workplace lactation support, part II: Working with the workplace. *Journal of Human Lactation,* 14(4): 321.
28. Kossek, E. E., and C. Ozeki. 1999. Bridging the work-family policy and productivity gap: A literature review. *Community, Work & Family.* 2(1): 7.
29. Lyness, K. S. et al. 1999. Work and pregnancy: Individual and organizational factors influencing organizational commitment, timing of maternity leave and return to work. *Sex Roles,* 41(7/8): 485.
30. Martocchio, J. J. 1992. The financial costs of absence decisions. *Journal of Management,* 18: 133.
31. Ballard, P. 1983. Breastfeeding for the working mother. *Issues in Comprehensive Pediatric Nursing,* 6: 249.
32. Cohen, R. et al. 1995. Comparison of maternal absenteeism and infant illness rates among breast-feeding and formula-feeding women in two corporations. *American Journal of Health Promotion,* 10: 148.
33. Auerbach, K. G., and E. Guss. 1984.
34. Auerbach, K. G. 1993. Maternal Employment and Breastfeeding. In K. G. Auerbach, and J. Riordan, eds. *Breastfeeding and Human Lactation.* Sudbury, MA: Jones & Bartlett. 401.

CHAPTER ELEVEN

HUMAN MILK FOR FRAGILE INFANTS

Lois D.W. Arnold, M.P.H., I.B.C.L.C.

Introduction

The literature on child survival is unequivocal about the importance of breastfeeding. While this body of literature tends to focus on the population of healthy infants born at term who then die of illness or conditions related to lack of breastfeeding, the importance of breastfeeding also holds true for the preterm infant and the infant who is sick at birth. Without breastfeeding or human milk, many infants and children die. For compromised infants the delivery of human milk may be a critical factor in whether the infant lives or dies.

Health professionals in "developed" countries may believe that the child survival literature only applies to countries with poor sanitation and contaminated water supplies. However, pockets of poverty with poor housing, poor sanitation, contaminated water supplies, and poor access to health care services can exist in the most affluent of nations, providing conditions that increase infant mortality disproportionately higher than in other areas of the same country. The United States is no exception to this fact.

It is a well-accepted premise in the United States that formulas (human milk substitutes) are "safe" and that infants and children do well on them. Formula is perceived as being "just as good as" human milk because we all know of individual formula-fed infants who are healthy, grow well, and sail through life with intelligence and charm. Yet study after study done on a *population* basis shows the long-term negative impact of formula feeding on health, resulting in increased health care costs as early as the first half year of life with additional costs well into adulthood.[1] This perception that an *individual* formula-fed infant will do well and suffer no ill effects from formula is the basis of problems for *populations* of preterm, ill or otherwise compromised fragile infants.

The Human Rights Framework for Breastfeeding and Human Milk for Sick Infants

Human rights usually involves a relationship between a government and its individual citizens and places responsibility on the government for taking an active role in many areas. In adopting human rights conventions, the United Nations places pressure on governments to be responsible for protecting the rights of its citizens. Countries who are signatory to these conventions are expected to honor them, with many countries using these conventions as a basis for legislation and regulation. This section relies heavily on the work of Bar-Yam, who has synthesized the material and placed breastfeeding and human milk in the United Nations conventions that address three categories of human rights: women's rights, children's rights, and the right to health and health care.[2]

While many of the conventions do not address breastfeeding directly, the right to health and well-being is addressed. Breastfeeding, therefore, fits into this framework both directly and indirectly as follows:

- **1948—Universal Declaration of Human Rights**
  Article 25: Everyone has a right to a standard of living that supports health and well-being of both the family and the individual. This includes adequate food. Mothers and children are identified as being entitled to special care and assistance. What better way to provide for health and well-being of families, mothers and children than to encourage and support breastfeeding and the provision of human milk to vulnerable infants?[3]
- **1976—International Covenant on Economic, Social and Cultural Rights**
  Article 10: This article protects the family as a fundamental unit of society and provides for both prenatal and postnatal protection for mothers. Countries are urged to adopt paid leave policies for working women and to provide special protections for all children.

Article 12: This article states that all have the right to the "highest attainable standard of physical and mental health." Countries need to take steps to lower infant mortality and ensure the healthy development of the child.[4]

Breastfeeding and human milk certainly fit into this convention well by providing child spacing benefits that protect the family as an economic unit. The relationship of breastfeeding and reduction in infant mortality rates and improvement in infant and child health outcomes needs no further elaboration in this chapter.

- **1981—Convention on the Elimination of All Forms of Discrimination Against Women**
  This convention recognizes that certain groups require special consideration.
  Article 5: The interests of the child have top priority. Citizens should be educated about maternity as a social function that protects society and that pregnant women and mothers should, therefore, be afforded special protection.
  Article 11: An extension of Article 5, this article states that discrimination against pregnant women in the workplace should be prevented and that women in the workplace should be protected against unsafe work practices and conditions.[5]

  "Breastfeeding" is understood to be part of "maternity" in this context, and should be protected also.[6]

Does "breastfeeding" mean merely consuming human milk or really being fed at the breast? If the baby/mother has the right to feed at the breast, then the mother has an obligation to do so. This requires government support. If the mother is unable to feed at the breast, then government is obligated to provide another source of breastfeeding; e.g. a wet nurse.

If the baby simply has the right to be fed human milk, again, mothers have an obligation to provide it. In its absence, governments then become obligated to provide human milk in some other way, such as a milk bank.

- **1989—Declaration and Convention on the Rights of the Child**
  Articles 3, 18: These articles state that the best interests of the child should always be primary. Article 18 specifies that governments should provide assistance to families through institutional and legislative support.[7]
  Article 24: This is the first place where breastfeeding is addressed directly (section 2e), stating that breastfeeding is an activity for the whole society. Mothers are not mandated to breastfeed, but governments are mandated to educate *all* mothers and parents so that they can make informed choices.[8]

These conventions clearly refer to all children and do not distinguish whether children are sick or well. What is inferred is that if a child is sick then the family and government clearly have obligations to remedy the situation where possible to "provide the highest attainable standard of physical and mental health." Breastfeeding and human milk, therefore, take on even greater importance for the fragile infant.

Policy Statements Encouraging the Use of Human Milk for Fragile Infants

UNICEF's GOBI Initiative

UNICEF has set forth a number of principles for improved child survival.[9] Dubbed "GOBI," these four principles were to become the foundation for health promotion and illness prevention programs throughout the world. The four principles are:

Growth

Oral rehydration

Breastfeeding

Immunization

Later additions to this campaign included the addition of Family Planning and Feeding. Despite the "arid" implications of the acronym, GOBI has been a fertile basis for improved infant and child health throughout the world.

Breastfeeding is the foundation of the campaign (even though it is third on the list), because it is an integral part of the other components. It provides the majority of infants with adequate growth for at least the first 6 months of life when practiced exclusively and is critical for continued optimal growth as supplements and complementary foods are added to the diet. Because human milk is 87 percent water, it provides adequate hydration even in the warmest climates and can prevent dehydration during bouts of diarrhea. The immune properties of colostrum and human milk provide early immunization and protection against disease to the nursing infant. Exclusive, frequent breastfeeding also promotes lactational amenorrhea and reduced fertility in the majority of women who practice exclusive breastfeeding for at least the first six months of the infant's life, providing a method of family planning that helps achieve optimal child spacing and protection of the health of the mother and the nursling who is still dependent on the mother for sustenance.[10]

WHO Feeding Hierarchy for Low Birth Weight Infants

Breastfeeding at the breast is the number one feeding option in the World Health Organization's hierarchy of infant feeding choices for infants who have the ability to breastfeed. For fragile and sick infants it may be that actual breastfeeding is impossible for a variety of reasons (e.g., gestational age, oromotor abnormalities) in which case the mother's fresh expressed milk becomes the first choice. Table 11.1 is a diagram of the hierarchy of feeding choices for low birth weight infants.[11] Publication of this hierarchy has become mired in international HIV politics, particularly in relation to the choices of fresh milk donated by a biologically unrelated mother (options 2 and 3). Countries such as the United States would not allow these two options to be used because the risk of disease transmission, in particular, HIV, outweighs the benefits of the fresh human milk. The schema represented in Table 11.2 would be more in keeping with United States policy. In developing countries where human milk substitutes carry a much higher risk of infant mortality than in a developed country, these two alternatives might be preferable because the risk of possible

TABLE 11.1   Milk for Low Birth Weight Babies
WHO hierarchy of feeding choices (version 1)

Best	Mother's own milk (fresh)	Helps bonding Helps establish lactation
	Donated fresh preterm milk	Good balance of nutrients (may need supplemental calcium and Vitamin D) Prevents infection Easily digested
	Donated fresh term mature milk	Prevents infection Easily digested, but lacks adequate protein Usually foremilk, so may lack adequate fat
	Pasteurized donated human milk	Easily digested HIV destroyed, but anti-infective factors partially lost
	Preterm formula	Correct nutrients, but not necessarily easily digestible No anti-infective properties More severe infections
Worst	Ordinary formula	Wrong balance of nutrients No anti-infective properties Less optimal growth and development

Adapted from F. Savage-King, personal communication with author, 1998.

TABLE 11.2   Milk for Low Birth Weight Babies
WHO hierarchy of feeding choices (version 2)

Best	Mother's own milk (fresh)	Helps bonding Helps establish lactation Good balance of nutrients (may need supplemental calcium and Vitamin D) Prevents infection Easily digested
	Pasteurized donated human milk	Easily digested, may lack adequate protein HIV, bacteria, and other viruses destroyed Anti-infective factors partially lost, but still protective against many diseases
	Preterm formula	Correct nutrients, but not necessarily easily digestible No anti-infective properties More severe infections
Worst	Ordinary formula	Wrong balance of nutrients No anti-infective properties Less optimal growth and development

Adapted from F. Savage-King, personal communication with author, 1998.

disease transmission and death from that disease is outweighed by the much higher risk of death from use of formula. Research by Coutsoudis has indicated that exclusive breastfeeding may convey much less risk of HIV transmission than mixed feeding.[12] These types of research questions need to be resolved before a firm policy, comfortable to all parties, can be developed.

WHO/UNICEF Baby-Friendly Hospital Initiative and Fragile Infants

The Baby-Friendly Hospital Initiative (BFHI), a joint WHO/UNICEF initiative established in 1991,[13] is also applicable to the fragile infant and older ill baby. Step 5 of the BFHI's *Ten Steps to Successful Breastfeeding* specifically states that mothers will be aided in the establishment and maintenance of lactation even when they must be separated from their infants.[14] Examples of acceptable separations are infants born prematurely who must be transferred to neonatal intensive care units or special care nurseries, infants born with birth anomalies that require additional medical support, and older infants and toddlers who are still breastfeeding but must be hospitalized for an illness or surgical procedure. Policies and procedures for ensuring that a mother is taught how to establish and/or maintain her milk supply during such separations should be in place (Step 1 of the *Ten Steps*), and all staff who come in contact with these mothers and their babies must be trained so that they can be supportive of the breastfeeding process and the use of human milk (Step 2).[15] Additionally, many neonatal intensive care units (NICU) and special care nurseries (SCN) rely on free supplies of special formulas, which may be considerably more expensive than the usual formulas. Within the WHO Code of Marketing[16] standards, all formulas should be paid for and, within the Baby-Friendly Hospital standards, used only when medically indicated (Step 6).[17]

Health care providers for this special group of babies should foster the development of and provide referrals to support groups, either in the hospital and/or in the community (mother-to-mother support groups, peer counseling, multidisciplinary teams) for specialized breastfeeding services and assistance (Step 10).[18] If such groups are not readily available in the community, it is the hospital's responsibility to establish support groups for breastfeeding mothers.[19]

U.S. Policy Statements

In 1997 the Work Group on Breastfeeding of the American Academy of Pediatrics published a positive statement about breastfeeding. Entitled "Breastfeeding and the Use of Human Milk," this statement makes it very clear that, "Human milk is the preferred feeding for all infants, including premature and sick newborns, with rare exceptions . . . . When direct breastfeeding is not possible, expressed human milk, fortified when necessary for the premature infant, should be provided."[20] The statement continues by saying "should hospitalization of the breastfeeding mother or infant be necessary, every effort should be made to maintain breastfeeding, preferably directly, or by pumping the breasts and feeding expressed breast milk, if necessary."[21] The United States Strategic Plan for Breastfeeding[22] and the Health and Human Services Blueprint[23] emphasize "comprehensive and seamless"[24] care for breastfeeding families.

In summary, numerous policy statements are available to support the concept that fragile babies need continued access to breastfeeding/ human milk. Intrinsic in these statements is the concept that feeding *at the breast* (= breastfeeding) is the ultimate goal, and that the delivery of a "product" (= human milk-feeding) is a stage along the way to full breastfeeding. As a population, premature and sick infants should eventually achieve the same breastfeeding rates as healthy term infants, even though they may take longer to achieve these rates.

Benefits of Human Milk for Fragile Infants

Defining the Fragile Infant

The fragile infant is any infant, newborn or otherwise, who has an illness or condition requiring special medical oversight. These illnesses or conditions may or may not be life threatening. Such illnesses and conditions include but are not limited to: prematurity and its related conditions, such as bronchopulmonary dysplasia, respiratory distress syndrome, and necrotizing enterocolitis; congenital anomalies, such as kidney malformations resulting in chronic renal insufficiency or failure, cardiac defects, clefts of the palate and lip, and gastroschisis; metabolic defects, also known as inborn errors of metabolism, and other genetic syndromes; conditions requiring surgery; infectious diseases requiring hospitalization; and immune deficiency syndromes. Fragile babies may or may not be hospitalized.

Fragile babies also include infants and children with terminal diseases or conditions. For these individuals, quality of life remaining is the issue.

Hospital Practices That Affect Breastfeeding and the Delivery of Human Milk

One of the important aspects of dealing with fragile infants, both premature and older ill infants, is to maintain the beneficial levels of many gut hormones. Somatostatin (SS) and cholecystokinin (CCK) are two gut peptides with opposite functions. SS inhibits various aspects of digestive function (pancreatic secretion, bile production and secretion, and production of other gut peptides), while CCK stimulates production and secretion of pancreatic juices and bile, stimulates peristalsis, and stimulates growth of the intestinal mucosa and pancreas.[25] From the work of Uvnäs-Moberg and others we know that when infants have high serum levels of the gut hormones gastrin and CCK they exhibit better growth by promoting insulin release and better utilization of nutrients.[26] Gastrin is produced in the gut in response to protein; and CCK, in response to fat. Both stimulate production of digestive components and growth of various digestive organs and tissues.

Sucking, feeding with species-specific milk, and peripheral nerve stimulation cause an increase in gastrin and CCK levels in the infant. Infants who are ill exhibit lower levels of gastrin and CCK. Necrotizing enterocolitis (NEC), for instance, adversely affects levels of gastrin in preterm infants.[27] Tornhage and colleagues report that SS levels are much higher in preterm infants and are inversely related to gestational age during the first several days of life.[28] Preterm infants fed their own mother's milk or donor milk through an NG tube had a rise in CCK levels from feeding and also had a significant increase when the infant was held in close contact with the mother. Breastfeeding infants showed a double-peak increase in CCK, and it is speculated that the first peak is due to the vagal nerve stimulation from the skin-to-skin contact and the second peak is caused by the food-stimulated release of CCK.[29] These authors suggest that for optimal release of growth-promoting GI hormones both the presence of food in the gut and enhanced sensory stimulation are needed.

Gastrin and CCK levels are also affected in the nursing mother through suckling. They rise during nursing and are thought to be associated with longer breastfeeding durations through a variety of mechanisms.[30] Hospital practices related to feeding and caring for small and sick infants can have an enormous impact on the levels of these two hormones and thus impact growth and metabolism of infants. Some of these practices, such as early initiation and frequency of breastfeeding, are also related to the optimal establishment of the mother's milk supply and to longer durations of breastfeeding. The practices under consideration for premature infants are early feeding and minimal enteral feedings; sucking on the "emptied" breast or a pacifier (= non-nutritive sucking); and skin-to-skin contact (= kangaroo care).

Early Feedings and Minimal Enteral Feeding

A review of enteral feeding practices can be found in Yu.[31] Some neonatologists feel that it is necessary to delay the start of enteral feedings in premature infants in order to avoid precipitating the onset of NEC. Berseth found that early-fed infants (fed on day 3–5 with Similac 20) exhibited more mature motor patterns (shorter transit times, less gastric residual, more frequent stooling) of the GI tract than late-fed babies (fed on day 10–14).[32] The early-fed babies also had higher serum levels of gastrin, indicating earlier ability to mount an insulin response and utilize nutrients. Berseth also notes that prolonged starvation promotes thinning of the intestinal mucosa with shortening of the villi (and consequent decrease in the surface area available for absorption of nutrients and production of digestive enzymes, leading to decreased digestive efficiency).[33] Unger and colleagues found that prolonged initial fasting or delay in initiation of enteral feeding was associated with a higher risk of nosocomial infection in a population of premature infants weighing less than 1000 grams at birth.[34] Lucas and Cole have shown that:

> "In infants fed breast milk timing of the first feed was not related to frequency of necrotising enterocolitis [NEC], but in formula-fed infants, delay in starting feeds was associated with a significant

reduction if enteral feeds were started on, for example, day 9 rather than day 2, the risk of necrotising enterocolitis was reduced three-fold."[35]

What the infant is fed thus makes a difference in early enteral feedings, with some neonatal units beginning enteral feedings of human milk within hours of the birth of the premature infant.

Additionally, early-fed infants have been shown in some studies to have better somatic growth. As Lucas points out, it is "fundamentally unphysiological to deprive an infant of any gestation of enteral feeding . . . ." because they have been swallowing amniotic fluid and "feeding" enterally in utero.[36] If the gut is deprived of enteral nutrition, atrophy results and gut peptide surges are abnormal.[37] When minimal enteral feedings are initiated early, these abnormal peptide surges do not occur, even when the infant is fed such small amounts that they are of no nutritional consequence (0.5 ml/feed).[38] With these peptide surges comes maturation of intestinal function and proliferation of the mucosal epithelium, desired occurrences if the infant is expected to grow. The consequences for the preterm infant are greater tolerance of enteral feedings, faster establishment of full enteral feeding and therefore less dependence on total parenteral nutrition (= hyperalimentation), decreased risk of NEC, possible decreased risk of allergy in families with a history of allergy (due to decreased gut permeability and faster closure of the gut with feeding, but reduction of risk is dependent on exclusivity of human milk feeding), decreased sepsis and nosocomial infections, and shorter hospital stays. In a review of randomized controlled trials, McClure found that disaccharidase activity in the gut was enhanced when trophic feeds of human milk were instituted, with considerably higher lactase activity at both the end of trophic feeds and up to 14 days after the introduction of larger amounts of enteral feedings. Also seen in the McClure review were elevations in postprandial plasma concentrations of gastrointestinal hormones (gastrin, etc.), increased blood flow in major gastrointestinal arteries, increased intestinal motility, reduction in the presence of pathogenic bacteria of the gut, increased milk tolerance, growth benefits in larger gains in weight and head circumference, reduction in duration of phototherapy, reduction in cases of sepsis, reduction in incidence of necrotizing enterocolitis, and a reduction in the length of hospital stay by 7–8 days. McClure stated that there is "currently no evidence of any adverse effects following trophic feeding."[39]

Schanler and colleagues, in comparing infants fed bovine-based fortifier plus human milk (FHM) versus preterm formula (PF), found that the FHM group was leaner than the PF group, even though it consumed considerably larger amounts of milk. The FHM group was healthier and had "significantly shorter hospitalization."[40] Schanler continues by saying that the smaller weight gain in the FHM group may be due to the excess amounts of magnesium, zinc, and copper in the fortifiers that may interfere with fat absorption, noticeably lower in the FHM group than the PF group. The bioactivity of the human milk lipid system may be affected by the addition of excess amounts of these minerals, and the fats themselves may be rendered less bioavailable.

For the newborn infant who has undergone GI surgery for a condition such as gastroschisis, early postoperative feedings of very small amounts may also be beneficial in promoting healing and establishing proper GI function by preventing hypertrophy from lack of enteral feeding.[41]

Sucking on the "Emptied" Breast and "Non-Nutritive Sucking"

Narayanan and colleagues describe this intervention as allowing the infant to suckle at the breast after as much milk as possible has been expressed.[42] The feeding was then given by tube while the infant was at the breast. Infants in this study were less than 1800 grams at birth and were unable to feed at the breast. As they became stronger, they were allowed to go to the breast. Initially, these infants merely mouthed the nipple, but could soon sustain sucking bursts alternating with rest periods. There were no episodes of choking with suckling at the "emptied" breast. The results of the study were that the intervention group had longer durations of exclusive and total breastfeeding than the control group. Milk production is stimulated by the infant suckling at the breast. The improved milk supply may encourage mothers to continue with exclusive breastfeeding longer, because they have more confidence in their ability to produce adequate milk. The long-term result of reduced infection would also be a benefit, especially in situations where the risk of infection is higher; e.g., lower socioeconomic groups.

Narayanan discusses the use of pacifiers to mature the suckling response and notes that the use of a pacifier in developing countries is contraindicated. In these situations the pacifier could further predispose a high-risk population to infection because of the inability to clean it properly, particularly after discharge from the hospital. However, the principle of sucking on a pacifier is to help induce a rise in gastrin and cholecystokinin and improve utilization of nutrients. In the United States the use of pacifiers is standard practice in many NICUs. A recent review of the literature on "non-nutritive suckling" (NNS) utilizing pacifiers, however, shows general lack of agreement among studies on whether there are benefits to pacifier use in the NICU with regard to sucking response, gastric emptying, and weight gain. Methodological flaws in the studies appeared to reduce the validity of results. The only positive association of pacifier use was found in relation to reduction in the length of hospital stay. Based on this review, the authors conclude "NNS cannot be currently recommended as a beneficial intervention."[43] It would appear to be better for both the mother's and the infant's gastrin and CCK levels (not to mention the mother's milk supply) if more of this non-nutritive sucking was conducted on the "empty" breast rather than on an inanimate object such as a pacifier.

Learning to suckle at the "empty" breast would also benefit the infant physiologically in that the frequently routine step of "bottling" a baby prior to learning to breastfeed could be avoided. Work by Meier shows that it is physiologically less stressful for preterm infants to breastfeed rather than bottle feed.[44] Fewer episodes of apnea and bradycardia are experienced when preterm infants are breastfed.

Skin-to-Skin Care

Initiating skin-to-skin (STS) care for preterm infants early in the intensive care experience results in significantly increased maternal milk volumes.[45] Those mothers practicing STS also reported that they were more relaxed and confident about breastfeeding and being able to meet their infant's needs. Whitelaw reports that mothers who practice STS breastfeed for longer durations.[46] Ludington-Hoe and others also report a physiological response between mother and infant when STS is practiced (maternal-neonatal thermal synchrony). Mothers physiologically assist in the thermoregulation of the infant, and infants experience better oxygenation, more stable heart rates, and less physiological stress during STS. In fact, the mother's breasts are exquisitely sensitive to the infant's temperature, and the mother can raise and lower her body temperature in response to the infant's temperature. Simultaneous measurement of maternal and infant temperatures showed that when the infant's temperature changed by as little as 0.2° C, the mother's temperature changed in the opposite direction by 1–2° C within one to two minutes.[47] Vasodilation of the breast in response to oxytocin release from suckling[48] or a conditioned response by the infant during STS may assist with this thermoregulation.

Föhe and colleagues showed that even infants weighing less than 1000 grams remained stable while STS and also showed a more efficient gas exchange. Physical positioning of the infant while STS may contribute to the effectiveness of STS. When positioned upright against the mother's chest, gravity may activate baroreceptors and cause an increase in heart rate, or the increase may be a direct result of increased body temperature from being STS. Massaging of the infant and rocking may also activate the central nervous system and cause an increase in heart rate. A decrease in respiratory rate may also partially be a function of the more upright positioning of an infant while STS. Weight of abdominal contents are shifted off the diaphragm and the ribcage moves more synchronously when the infant is in an upright position. Because infants also sleep more quietly when STS with their mothers, this may also result in more "tranquil" respiration and a higher oxygen saturation.[49]

Breastfeeding the Older Infant and STS

Increased STS contact and opportunities to nurse in the older hospitalized baby also have value. For older babies or toddlers who have undergone surgery or who are hospitalized for some reason, STS can be beneficial in that it will help to lower somatostatin levels and increase gastrin and CCK levels, improving the ability of the ill infant to obtain ideal nutrition through peripheral nerve stimulation. Furthermore, STS and breastfeeding for the older infant may contribute enormously toward comforting a baby in pain; the physiological stress of dealing with the pain may be reduced considerably with STS and breastfeeding. Many mothers have experienced the calming effect of STS and breastfeeding in infants and toddlers who have sustained injuries in common childhood accidents, such as scraped knees. Evidence now points to the efficacy of STS as a "potent intervention against the pain experienced" during many hospital procedures, such as heel sticks in newborns.[50] Lawrence states:

> The infant who requires surgery or rehospitalization can and should be breastfed postoperatively in most cases . . . The infant who is hospitalized is already traumatized by the separation, the strange surroundings and the people, and the underlying discomfort of the disease process itself. If the infant is to be fed orally, feeding should be at the breast as much as possible . . . The infant should not be subjected to the added trauma of being weaned from the breast when the infant needs the security and intimacy of nursing most . . . The medical profession needs to be aware of this infant and mother and their special needs for support . . . The pediatrician should assume the advocacy role. The parents should not have to fight for the right to maintain breastfeeding.[51]

Popper points out that many ill toddlers and infants will continue to breastfeed even when they refuse other food and drink that they may have been eating previous to the surgery or illness.[52] Unfamiliar foods in the hospital setting may be difficult to digest. Breastfeeding thus continues to have great nutritional significance in the older baby or toddler who cannot tolerate other foods. It also provides important immune factors protecting the infant from nosocomial infections. Breastfeeding may also help to maintain a more normal routine for babies and toddlers, and in so doing contributes to an environment in which they can better cope with discomfort.

Recommendations

In one informal survey of breastfeeding mothers of infants with congenital heart disease, mothers were asked to identify institutional barriers to successful breastfeeding. Obstacles which they identified were negative attitudes of health care providers, persistent questions about whether the infant was "getting enough" milk, lack of privacy for breastfeeding and/or expressing milk, lack of adequate pumping facilities and pumps when they were separated from their infants, and inconsistent recommendations from health care providers.[53] Other studies have found a strong correlation with maternal perception of inadequate milk supply as being a major factor in weaning of preterm infants.[54]

The use of a mother's own milk and/or breastfeeding needs to be protected, promoted, and supported unequivocally in the neonatal intensive care setting, the pediatric intensive care setting, and any other pediatric unit which might have admissions of breastfed children. To achieve this goal, attitudes and philosophies among various disciplines in the medical profession need to be examined carefully, as seen in the Lambert and Watters survey.[55] This is an extremely important component of providing care for this population of infants and children, and until attitudes change, breastfeeding promotion, protection, and support will not succeed in this setting. The following misconceptions and attitudes are prevalent today and are barriers to successful breastfeeding and the use of human milk in the NICU:

- *Human milk is inadequate nutritionally and deficient calorically.* Many physicians and dietitians believe this is so because they cannot measure its components. Even if they could measure the milk, they would have to do so at each feeding because of the dynamism and variation in milk composition from one point in time to the next. What we do know is that despite the slower growth of infants fed human milk when compared to infants fed formula, other positive outcomes such as improved health can be more important and outweigh (so to speak!) the slower weight gain.[56] There is no reason to substitute a formula when human milk can be fortified to achieve other favorable outcomes. Choice of the type of fortifier used may also have an impact on duration of lactation, with parental preference for a powdered fortifier being positively associated with longer breastfeeding durations in very low birth weight (VLBW) infants.[57]

- *Human milk causes illness in infants because it has bacteria in it.* In NICUs a mother's milk may be blamed first for an infant's illness. In some units, all milk is tested bacteriologically before it can be fed to an infant, implying that mothers and their milk are dirty. Yet anecdotal observations of twins receiving the same milk show that individual babies do not respond the same way to the same feedings. One twin may get sick while the other thrives, yet nothing about the feeding is different. Still, the milk gets the blame when alternative causes should be considered first (e.g., something intrinsic in the twin's condition that predisposes him to that illness or poor infection control procedures on the part of the staff feeding the infant). One Canadian study showed clearly that sepsis was not related to bacteria the infant was exposed to through feeding, as all cases of sepsis were caused by organisms that the infant was colonized with prior to feeding.[58]

- *Human milk has no value after the infant starts solids and complementary foods.* Many care providers feel that human milk has no value beyond the first several months of life. The AAP statement should help in changing this perception.[59] It is especially important to correct this misconception if the ill or fragile baby refuses to eat anything else, as indicated in Popper.[60]

- *Mothers cannot be trusted to provide clean milk for their babies.* It has been observed that some hospitals do not trust mothers to provide milk except when it is expressed in the hospital setting. Hospitals may refuse to feed milk expressed by mothers at home, feeding only what had been expressed under supervision of the hospital staff. This means that most infants will be fed formula, because mothers live several hours away from the tertiary care facility and can only express in the hospital during visits as few as once or twice a week.

- *The baby belongs to the hospital team, not the parents, and the hospital staff is all-knowing and RIGHT in what it knows!* This attitude is expressed in case histories from Popper.[61] The implicit threat is that if the mother does not do things the way the staff wants her to, she will be reported to Children's Protective Services and her custody rights will be questioned/terminated. The mother who asks questions and defends doing what is best for her baby—expressing her milk or breastfeeding—should not be labeled a trouble-maker by the staff. Barriers to participation in the baby's care and defense mechanisms used by mothers in the intensive care unit are described by Fenwick and colleagues and Hurst.[62]

To combat these prejudices and attitudes, changes are needed at the national level. First, training should be better across the board in breastfeeding management and lactation physiology in medical schools, nursing schools, midwifery programs, and nutrition degree programs. This basic knowledge should be required of all students no matter what specialty they may focus on later in their careers. Breast-feeding impacts women and infants in all ages and stages; even as geri-atric specialists we need to understand the impact of breastfeeding on improving bone mineral density and reducing the risk of hip fracture so that we can encourage ourselves, our neighbors, our clients, our wives, our siblings, and our grandchildren to breastfeed.

Second, this training should be evidence-based and continued in residency programs, practicums, and internships. Specialty conferences should devote offerings to the specifics of breastfeeding management and lactation physiology and the benefits to specific groups of infants and children. Currently, textbooks on infant nutrition and nutrition of the young child with illnesses or chronic conditions may fail to even mention breastfeeding, illustrating the depth of the lack of knowledge.

Third, the Joint Commission on Healthcare Accreditation should consider hospitals with neonatal and pediatric services in terms of the quality of policies and procedures regarding the use of human milk.

Fourth, a parameter that might be useful not only to change attitudes but also to assess individual babies is a growth chart for preterm infants that is not based on intrauterine accretion rates. Because these infants are no longer in utero, it may not be fair to expect them to grow at the same rate as an intrauterine fetus, because conditions are not the same and the mother is no longer "subsidizing" the infant's metabolic needs. It can be argued that the intrauterine accretion rates are the only measures we have, and therefore we must continue using them, inade-quate though they may be. If they are inadequate for the situation, per-haps they are doing more harm than good, and infant growth patterns are being judged unfairly by a standard which may or may not be accurate or beneficial in the long term. Focus needs to be placed on pediatric outcome measures (the macro-picture) rather than on how many milligrams of something an infant got at each feeding (the micro-picture). At the risk of oversimplifying, feeding the premature and sick infant has become a game of number crunching, weighing and mea-suring everything to the exclusion of using human milk or using it only in token fashion because it does not fit into this numbers game well.

At the local level, specific policies need to be implemented in both NICU, SCN, and pediatric settings. These policies and practices are de-lineated below. In all cases where the infant cannot nurse immediately after birth and mother and baby must be separated:

- The mother should be educated and counseled about the impor-tance of her milk for her infant and that supplying her own milk is a medical necessity for her infant.
- The multidisciplinary team responsible for the care of the mother and infant should give consistent information and assist the

mother in beginning to express her milk as soon as she is physically capable.

- Policies and procedures should be in place for the following:
  - Helping a mother express and maintain a milk supply (frequency of pumping was predictive of adequate milk supply by weeks 4 and 5)[63]
  - Storing and handling mothers' milk in the hospital setting to minimize contamination[64]
  - Delivering human milk to the infant in ways which minimize nutrient losses[65]
  - Encouraging and initiating skin-to-skin care as soon as possible (positively associated with increased milk volumes)[66]
  - Preventing accidental use of another mother's milk
  - Initiating early enteral feedings with full strength human milk
  - Using undiluted human milk
  - Beginning fortification of feedings (when and how), including what type of fortification and research-based protocols for other methods of "beefing up" milk, such as feeding high-fat milk, infrared analysis of milk for individualized fortification, ultrasonic homogenization, etc.[67]
  - Demand feeding rather than feeding human milk on a schedule that may not reflect actual gastric emptying times and the low residuals left in the gut; scheduled feedings may be depriving infants of needed nutrition[68]
  - Using tube feeding at the breast (so the infant learns to associate the feeling of fullness with being at the breast) and recognizing that, for developmentally ready infants, the learning curve for full breastfeeding may be as long as three weeks[69]
  - Recognizing that infants may be ready to breastfeed much earlier than their gestational age indicates[70]
  - Using alternative feeding methods other than bottles to transition to the breast when oral feedings are indicated[71]

For the breastfeeding baby or toddler who is rehospitalized for illness or surgery, many of the same recommendations for policies and procedures apply.

- Providing adequate facilities and pumps for expression to all mothers of hospitalized infants for the occasions when they may not be able to breastfeed directly
- Ensuring that protocols are in place relating to the proper storage, handling, fortification, and delivery of human milk feedings to the infant who is unable to breastfeed[72]
- Developing protocols allowing for breastfeeding within two hours prior to surgery on an "emptied" breast to assist in keeping the

infant calm; similar protocols can be developed for the recovery period if actual breastfeeding intake must be restricted[73]

- Adopting the principles of the *Ten Steps to Successful Breastfeeding* in pediatric units, adapting as needed to fit the needs of the older nursing population.
- Providing staff support for breastfeeding mothers through a multi-disciplinary team that provides consistent information and proactive assistance

Summary

A premature or sick infant has the right to be fed his or her own mother's milk in most circumstances. Compelling physiological reasons exist why human milk is the BEST for most infants. Likewise, compelling reasons exist for changing hospital policies and procedures to accommodate the routine use of human milk and/or breastfeeding in the intensive care nursery or pediatric unit. Furthermore, every infant who begins life being fed expressed human milk has the right to learn how to breastfeed. The period of hospitalization and use of expressed human milk should be thought of as a pause in the journey along the road to full breastfeeding. Breastfeeding is the right of every infant whether or not a medical condition exists at birth that might delay the establishment of breastfeeding. For the woman who delivers a preterm infant and cannot immediately feed directly at the breast, the ultimate goal should be for a breastfeeding dyad that continues to breastfeed long after hospital discharge. Mothers of preterm and sick infants also have the right to have long-term breastfeeding outcomes similar to those women who deliver at term.

In order to achieve these long-term breastfeeding outcomes, hospital policies need to change radically. They should encourage skin-to-skin contact, early enteral feedings, as little separation of mother and infant as possible, the use of expressed human milk in preference to special formulas, and support in the hospital and in the community for mothers going through a difficult period trying to mechanically establish and maintain a milk supply under stressful conditions.

References and Notes

1. Ball, T. M., and A. L. Wright. 1999. Health care costs of formula-feeding in the first year of life. *Pediatrics* 103(4): 870.
Pettitt, D. et al. 1997. Breastfeeding and incidence of NIDDM in Pima Indians. *The Lancet* 350: 166.

Davis, M. K. et al.1988. Infant feeding and childhood cancer. *Lancet* August 13: 365.

Freudenheim, D. 1994. Exposure to breastmilk in infancy and the risk of breast cancer. *Epidem.* 5: 324.

2. Bar-Yam, N. 2000. *The Right to Breast: Breastfeeding and Human Rights.* Health Education Associates Inc.: Sandwich, MA.

3. Bar-Yam, N. 2000. 32.

4. Ibid.

5. Ibid., 34.

6. Ibid., 35.

7. Ibid., 37–38.

8. Ibid., 39–40.

9. UNICEF/WHO/UNESCO/UNFPA. 1993. Facts for Life. Oxfordshire, UK: P & LA.

10. Labbok, M. et al. 1994. *Guidelines: Breastfeeding, Family Planning, and the Lactational Amenorrhea Method—LAM.* Washington DC: Institute of Reproductive Health.

11. F. Savage-King. 1998. Personal communication with author.

12. Coutsoudis, A. et al. 1999. Influence of infant-feeding patterns on early mother-to-child transmission of HIV-1 in Durban, South Africa: A prospective cohort study. *The Lancet* 354: 471.

13. Grant, J. P. 1991. Joint WHO-UNICEF letter to Heads of State/Government on the Baby Friendly Hospital Initiative (BFHI). Executive Directive CF/EXD-IC/1991-028, 26 September.

Grant, J. P. 1991. Baby-Friendly Hospital Initiative. Executive Directive CF/EXD-IC/1991-028.add, 30 December.

14. Step 5 of the Ten Steps to Successful Breastfeeding is "Show mothers how to breastfeed, and how to maintain lactation even if they should be separated from their infants." UNICEF and World Health Organization. 1989. *Protecting, Promoting and Supporting Breast-Feeding: The Special Role of Maternity Services.* Geneva: WHO, iv.

15. Step 1 of the Ten Steps to Successful Breastfeeding is "Have a written breast-feeding policy that is routinely communicated to all health care staff." Ibid.

Step 2 of the Ten Steps to Successful Breastfeeding is "Train all health care staff in skills necessary to implement this policy." Ibid.

16. World Health Organization 1994. International Code of Marketing of Breast-Milk Substitutes, adopted May 1981. In Armstrong, H.C., & Sokol: *The International Code of Marketing of Breast-Milk Substitutes: What it Means for Mothers and Babies World-Wide.* Raleigh, NC: ILCA, 24–28.

17. Step 6 of the Ten Steps to Successful Breastfeeding is "Give newborn infants no food or drink other than breast milk, unless *medically* indicated."

18. Step 10 of the Ten Steps to Successful Breastfeeding is "Foster the establishment of breast-feeding support groups and refer mothers to them on discharge from the hospital or clinic." Ibid.

19. United States Committee for UNICEF and Wellstart International. 1998. *The U.S. Baby-Friendly Hospital Initiative: Guidelines and Evaluation*

Criteria for Hospital/Birthing Center Level Implementation. Washington, DC: Author.

20. American Academy of Pediatrics, Work Group on Breastfeeding. 1997. Breastfeeding and the use of human milk. *Pediatrics* 100, 1036.

21. Ibid., 1037.

22. United States Breastfeeding Committee. 2001. *Breastfeeding in the United States: A National Agenda.* Rockville MD: United States Department of Health and Human Services, Health Resources and Services Administration, Maternal and Child Health Bureau.

23. United States Department of Health and Human Services. 2000. *HHS Blueprint for Action on Breastfeeding.* Office of Women's Health, United States Department of Health and Human Services: Washington, DC.

24. United States Breastfeeding Committee. 2001. Objective C, Strategy 1. 8.

25. Tornhage, C. J. et al. 1998. Plasma somatostatin and cholecystokinin levels in response to feeding in preterm infants. *J. Pediatr. Gastroenterol. Nutr.* 27: 199.

26. Uvnäs-Moberg, K., and J. Winberg. 1989. Role for sensory stimulation in energy economy of mother and infant with particular regard to the gastrointestinal endocrine system. Chapter 7 in *Textbook of Gastroenterology and Nutrition in Infancy,* E. Lebenthal, ed. Raven Press Ltd: New York. 53–62.

27. Gounaris, A. et al. 1997. Gut hormone concentrations in preterm infants with necrotizing enterocolitis. *Acta. Paediatr.* 86: 762.

28. Tornhage, C. J. et al. 1997. Plasma somatostatin and cholecystokinin levels in sick preterm infants during their first six weeks of life. *Acta. Paediatr.* 86: 847.

29. Tornhage, C. J. et al. 1998. Plasma somatostatin and cholecystokinin levels in response to feeding in preterm infants. *J. Pediatr. Gastroenterol. Nutr.* 27: 199.

30. Uvnäs-Moberg, K., and J. Winberg. 1989. 58.

31. Yu, V. Y. H. 1999. Enteral feeding in the preterm infant. *Early Hum. Devel.* 56: 89.

32. Berseth, C. L. 1992. Effect of early feeding on maturation of the preterm infant's small intestine. *J. Pediatr.* 120: 947.
See also: Schanler, R. J. et al. 1999. Feeding strategies for premature infants: Randomized trial of gastrointestinal priming and tube-feeding method. *Pediatrics* 103: 434.

33. Berseth, C. L. 1995. Minimal enteral feedings. *Clins. Perinatol.* 22: 195.

34. Unger, A. et al. 1986. Nutritional practices and outcome of extremely premature infants. *Amer. J. Dis. Child.* 140: 1027.

35. Lucas, A., and T. J. Cole. 1990. Breast milk and neonatal necrotising enterocolitis. *The Lancet* 336: 1522.

36. Lucas, A. 1993. Enteral nutrition. Chap. 14 in *Nutritional Needs of the Preterm Infant: Scientific Basis and Practical Guidelines.* Tsang, R. et al., eds. Williams & Wilkins: Baltimore. 219.
Lucas, A. et al. 1996. Randomized outcome trial of human milk fortification and developmental outcome in preterm infants. *Amer. J. Clin. Nutr.* 64: 142.

37. Lucas, A. et al. 1983. Metabolic and endocrine consequences of depriving preterm infants of enteral nutrition. *Acta. Paediatr. Scand.* 72: 245.

38. Lucas, A. et al. 1986. Gut hormones and "minimal enteral feeding." *Acta. Paediatr. Scand.* 75: 719.
Lucas, A. 1993. 209.

39. McClure, R. J. 2001. Trophic feeding of the preterm infant. *Acta. Paediatr. Suppl.* 436: 19.

40. Schanler, R. J. et al. 1999. Feeding strategies for premature infants: beneficial outcomes of feeding fortified human milk versus preterm formula. *Pediatrics* 103: 1150, 1155.

41. Lucas, A. et al. 1986.
Rangecroft, L. et al. 1978. A comparison of the feeding of the postoperative newborn with banked breast-milk or cow's-milk feeds. *J. Pediatr. Surg.* 13: 11.

42. Narayanan, I. et al. 1991. Sucking on the "emptied" breast: Non-nutritive sucking with a difference. *Arch. Dis. Child.* 66: 241.

43. Premji, S. S., and B. Paes. 2000. Gastrointestinal function and growth in premature infants: Is non-nutritive sucking vital? *J. Perinatol.* 1: 46.

44. Meier, P. 1988. Bottle and breastfeeding: Effects on transcutaneous oxygen pressure and temperature in preterm infants. *Nurs. Res.* 37: 35.

45. Hurst, N. M. et al. 1997. Skin-to-skin holding in the neonatal intensive care unit influences maternal milk volume. *J. Perinatol.* 17: 213.

46. Whitelaw, A. 1986. Skin-to-skin contact in the care of very low birthweight babies. *Mat. Child. Hlth.* 7: 242.
Whitelaw, A. et al. 1988. Skin-to-skin contact for very low birthweight infants and their mothers. *Arch. Dis. Child.* 63: 1377.
See also: Ludington-Hoe, S. M., and J. Y. Swinth. 1996. Developmental aspects of kangaroo care. *JOGNN* 25: 691.

47. Ludington-Hoe, S. M. et al. 1994. Kangaroo care: Research results, and practice implications and guidelines. *Neonatal Network* 13: 19.

48. Uvnäs-Moberg, K., and J. Winberg. 1989. 53.

49. Föhe, K. et al. 2000. Skin-to-skin contact improves gas exchange in premature infants. *J. Perinatol.* 5: 311.

50. Gray, L. et al. 2000. Skin-to-skin contact is analgesia in healthy newborns. *Pediatrics* 105: e14.
[http://www.pediatrics.org/cgi/content/full/105/1/e14].

51. Lawrence, R. A. 1999. Breastfeeding the infant with a problem. Chap. 14 in Lawrence RA & Lawrence RM, *Breastfeeding: A Guide for the Medical Profession,* 5th edition. 497.

52. Popper, B. K. 1998. Unit 1, Lactation Consultant Series Two. *The Hospitalized Nursing Baby.* La Leche League International: Schaumburg, IL.

53. Lambert, J. M., and N. E. Watters. 1998. Breastfeeding the infant/child with a cardiac defect: An informal survey. *J. Hum. Lact.* 14: 151.

54. Hill, P. D. et al. 1995. Delayed initiation of breastfeeding the preterm infant. *J. Perinat. Neonat. Nurs.* 9: 10.

55. Ibid.

56. Schanler, R. J. et al. 1999.

57. Fenton, T. et al. 2000. Breast milk supplementation for preterm infants: Parental preferences and postdischarge lactation duration. *Am. J. Perinatol.* 17: 329.

58. Law, B. J. et al. 1989. Is ingestion of milk-associated bacteria by premature infants fed raw human milk controlled by routine bacteriologic screening? *J. Clin. Microbiol.* 27: 1560.

59. American Academy of Pediatrics, Work Group on Breastfeeding. 1997. Breastfeeding and the use of human milk. *Pediatrics* 100: 1035.

60. Popper, B. K. 1998. Unit 1, Lactation Consultant Series Two. *The Hospitalized Nursing Baby.* La Leche League International: Schaumburg, IL.

61. Ibid.

62. Fenwick, J. et al. Struggling to mother: A consequence of inhibitive nursing interactions in the neonatal nursery. *J. Perinat. Neonat. Nurs.* 15: 49.
Hurst, I. 2001. Mothers' strategies to meet their needs in the newborn intensive care nursery. *J. Perinat. Neonat. Nurs.* 15: 65.

63. Hill, P. D. et al. 1999. Effects of pumping style on milk production in mothers of non-nursing preterm infants. *J. Hum. Lact.* 15: 209.

64. Arnold, L. D. W. 1999. *Recommendations for Collection, Storage and Handling of a Mother's Milk for Her Own Infant in the Hospital Setting.* 3rd edition. Human Milk Banking Association of North America, Inc: Denver, CO.

65. Ibid.
Greer, F. R. et al. 1984. Changes in fat concentration of human milk during delivery by intermittent bolus and continuous mechanical pump infusion. *J. Pediatr.* 105: 745.
Hamosh, M. 1994. Digestion in the premature infant: The effects of human milk. *Sem. Perinatol.* 18: 485.
Kaempf, J. 1991. Techniques of enteral feeding in the preterm infant. Ch. 14 in *Neonatal Nutrition and Metabolism.* Hay, W.W., ed. Mosby Year Book: St. Louis, MO. 335.
Lucas, A. 1993. 217.

66. Hill, P. D. et al. 1999. Effects of pumping style on milk production in mothers of non-nursing preterm infants. *J. Hum. Lact.* 15: 209.

67. Hamosh, M. 1994. Digestion in the premature infant: The effects of human milk. *Sem. Perinatol.* 18: 485.
Michaelsen, K. F. et al. 1988. Infrared analysis for determining macronutrients in human milk. *J. Pediatr. Gastroent. Nutr.* 7: 229.
Rayol, M. R. S. et al. 1993. Feeding premature infants banked human milk homogenized by ultrasonic treatment. *J. Pediatr.* 123: 985.

68. Hamosh recommends avoiding use of restricted volumes of milk. Hamosh, M. 1994. Digestion in the premature infant: The effects of human milk. *Sem. Perinatol.* 18: 485.

69. Wheeler, J. L. et al. 1999. Promoting breastfeeding in the neonatal intensive care unit. *Breastfeed. Rev* 7: 15.

70. Nyqvist, K. H. et al. 1999. The development of preterm infants' breastfeeding behavior. *Early Hum. Devel.* 55: 247.

71. For a protocol without bottles, see Stine, M. J. 1990. Breastfeeding the premature newborn: A protocol without bottles. *J. Hum. Lact.* 6: 167. For studies on safety and efficacy of cup feeding see Marinelli, K., and V. Dodd. 1998. Safety of cup vs. bottle feedings in premature breastfed infants [abstract]. *ABM News and Views* 4: 23.
Howard, C. R. et al. 1998. Physiologic stability of infants during cup and bottle feeding [abstract]. *ABM News and Views* 4: 23.

72. Arnold, L. D. W. 1999.

73. Lawrence, R. A. 1999. Breastfeeding the infant with a problem. Chapter 14 in Lawrence, R. A. and R. M. Lawrence, *Breastfeeding: A Guide for the Medical Profession,* 5th edition. 443.

CHAPTER TWELVE

USING BANKED DONOR MILK
IN CLINICAL SETTINGS

Lois D. W. Arnold, M.P.H., I.B.C.L.C.

Defining Donor Milk Banking

As the term implies, banked donor milk is milk that a mother collects (in excess of what her own baby needs) and gives to an organized milk banking entity. This ensures the safety of the milk through donor screening, milk bacteriology, and pasteurization. Processed donor milk is dispensed by the milk bank on prescription to infants, children, and the occasional adult with specific medical or nutritional needs for human milk.

Donor milk banking is recognized in the hierarchy of feeding choices developed by the World Health Organization (see Tables 11.1 and 11.2). In a 1980 joint resolution, WHO and UNICEF refer to banked donor milk as the "first alternative" when a mother's own milk is unavailable.[1] In a later statement, donor milk was listed as an acceptable alternative when the biological mother tested positive for HIV.[2] Donor milk fits the FDA's definition of an "orphan product or biological" because it is used to serve a population of under 200,000 individuals each year with specific medical needs for banked donor milk.[3] Innovative uses for donor milk, described later in this chapter, could also place it in a category of "alternative" medicine or therapy. Donor milk is much more than nutrition; it is a tissue transplant, a medicine, and a valuable part of the health care system.

Processing and Quality Control

A flow chart has been developed in Figure 12.1 for visualization of the donor milk banking process.[4] Many mothers collect milk in an ongoing fashion, donating over a period of weeks or months. Other mothers may find that they have expressed and stored much more than their infants will use and decide to make a one-time donation. In some cases, mothers who have preterm infants who die or infants with birth anomalies incompatible with life will donate the milk they have accumulated helping the mother to grieve for her loss and find some good in a heart-wrenching situation.

Guidelines for operating donor milk banks have been developed in the United States by the Human Milk Banking Association of North America, Inc. (HMBANA), in consultation with representatives of the Food and Drug Administration (FDA) and the Centers for Disease Control and Prevention (CDC). Individual milk banks comply with the guidelines on a voluntary basis. These guidelines, reviewed and revised annually, detail the

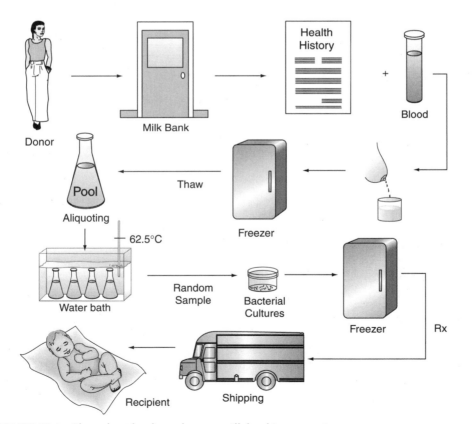

FIGURE 12.1   Flow chart for donor human milk banking operations

screening and processing which must occur before donor milk is dispensed.[5] Guidelines are written in general terms so that milk banks can still operate practically within their own resource constraints while still operating safely.[6] Donor milk banks in the United States must also comply with guidelines developed by the United States Public Health Service for tissue and organ transplant banks.[7] Since human milk in its raw form contains live cells and is capable of transmitting various diseases, both bacterial and viral, banked donor milk which goes to biologically unrelated recipients must be classified as a tissue transplant as well as a food.

All donors must undergo a thorough screening before the milk can be used. An intensive verbal health history is taken, and mothers may be excluded from donating at the time if they do not meet certain criteria. Additionally they are serum-screened for certain viral diseases, including HIV (Figure 12.2). Both the mother's and the infant's primary care provider are requested to certify that the prospective donor and her infant are in good health. (Underlying causes of death are examined on an individual basis when the infant has died or the donor has had a fetal demise.)

Although demographics have never been collected and analyzed, donors are predominantly Caucasian, middle-class, educated women. Between 1990 and 1995, 1,226 donors were serum screened by six U.S. milk banks. Of the tests listed in Figure 12.2, only three of the tests (HTLV, Hepatitis B, Hepatitis C) had any donors who tested positive. Of the 1,226 donors tested, only 14 showed positive tests, and on retesting only three of these were true positive tests, as shown in Figure 12.3.

- HIV-1 and HIV-2 antibody and antigen
- Human T-Cell Leukemia Virus (HTLV) antibody
- Hepatitis B surface antigen
- Hepatitis C antibody
- Syphilis

FIGURE 12.2   Serological tests for donors—2001

HTLV antibody
    7 reactive tests, 6 false positive, 1 indeterminate
Hepatitis B surface antigen
    1 reactive test
Hepatitis C antibody
    6 reactive tests, 4 false positive, 2 true reactive
Total reactive tests = 14 (1.1% incidence)
Total true reactive tests = 3 (0.24% incidence)

FIGURE 12.3   Donor screening results, 1990 through 1994. (n = 1,226 donors screened)[8]

Processing of the milk in the United States is done in constant-temperature water baths. Milks from several different donors are pooled (to average the composition), then aliquoted to 2- or 4-ounce bottles with watertight lids. These bottles are then submerged in the water bath, brought to temperature (either 56° C [heat treatment] or 62.5° C [Holder pasteurization]) and held there for thirty minutes. Two studies show that HIV is destroyed by heat treatment at these temperatures.[9] The heat reaction is stopped by plunging the bottles into an ice slurry. Bottles are then labeled and frozen. Some milk banks test the milk for bacteria before pasteurization as a means of quality control of the donor's collection methods; others test only after the milk has undergone processing. Processed milk may not be dispensed unless there are no bacterial colony forming units present (0 CFU/ml).

Banked donor milk is dispensed only on prescription.[10] Milk is shipped frozen to the recipient family on an outpatient basis or is shipped frozen directly to the hospital. Some hospitals have standing orders for a specific number of ounces to be delivered each week. Banked donor milk can be delivered within twenty-four hours of receiving the prescription. Milk can be shipped anywhere in the country from any of the milk banks in the United States, and the recipient family is usually charged for the shipping costs.

Benefits of Banked Donor Milk

The benefits of using banked donor milk are most obvious for the recipient, but benefits accrue to the family of the recipient, the donor, and society as well.

The Recipient

For the recipient, the ease of digestibility of human milk is of paramount importance because there is less metabolic stress. For example, if the preterm infant spends less energy digesting its food, there is more energy available for breathing, for accretion of tissues, and for growth in general. The unique composition of milk and its species-specificity also play a role in the reduction of metabolic stress as well as in the proper and desired growth and maturation of tissues and organs. For the infant whose GI tract may have been damaged by human milk substitutes, repair and healing is accelerated when banked human milk with its growth factors is introduced to the infant's diet. Infants often stop screaming in pain when donor milk is introduced, and constipation, GI bleeding, or diarrhea are resolved frequently within hours of starting the use of donor milk. Adults with GI tract problems also benefit from the healing nature of banked donor milk in conditions such as reflux and ulcerative colitis.[11]

Immunological benefits are also present for the recipient, none of which human milk substitutes or other foods can replicate.[12] For a preterm infant with an immature immune system, this added protection may mean that the infant has fewer episodes of being taken off oral feedings. As public health experts know, when nutrition is compromised, the immune system is compromised also; the infant has less resistance to disease, and any illness in turn may further compromise nutritional status in a cycle which may ultimately result in the death of the infant. See Figure 12.4. For the adult recipient, the banked donor milk may provide an immune substance for which the recipient has a deficiency (e.g. IgA).[13]

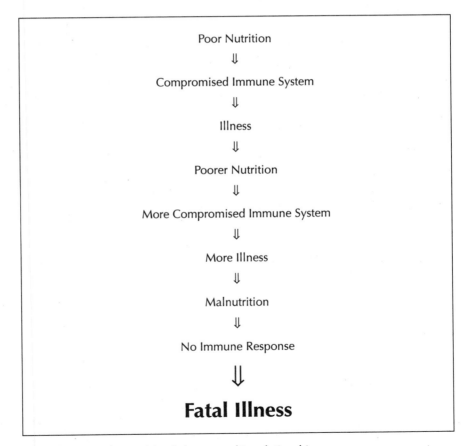

Poor Nutrition

⇓

Compromised Immune System

⇓

Illness

⇓

Poorer Nutrition

⇓

More Compromised Immune System

⇓

More Illness

⇓

Malnutrition

⇓

No Immune Response

⇓

Fatal Illness

FIGURE 12.4   The nutrition/infant mortality relationship

The Recipient's Family

For the family of the recipient, one major benefit is that the infant's discomfort and pain is relieved. Many parents report that the infant on donor milk is less fussy and spends less time being uncomfortable and complaining about being in pain, even in situations where the infant has been known to have a fatal condition.[14] For parents, this easing of infant discomfort relieves their own anguish and stress. Other parents of recipients find that the availability of donor milk offered a sense of security; if the mother's own supply ran low, there was appropriate backup for her own milk supply.

Society

In a larger community setting, the availability and frequent use of donor milk speaks volumes about the importance of human milk/breastfeeding to the health and well-being of infants. The message that comes with this use is: "We think that breastfeeding/human milk is so important to the well-being of our patients that we will use donor milk if you cannot supply your own milk." This is extremely positive public press for the benefits of breastfeeding and the medical necessity for providing human milk to fragile infants.

The Donor

For the donor there is a wonderful feeling of having done something special. Not only is she providing something superlative for her own baby, she is doing something for another infant in sharing the wealth. She truly makes a difference on a much broader scale. This gives donors, especially those who donate over a period of months, what might be called the "warm fuzzies." It makes them feel good, and who doesn't want to keep a "feel good" feeling going? Mothers who lose infants may find that donating the accumulated supply helps to initiate the grieving process. Continuing to express over a period of weeks for a milk bank after a fetal demise helps women to feel like mothers, even when they have no baby.

Drawbacks of Donor Milk

One of the biggest objections to banked donor milk among prescribers arises from the mistaken belief that all the beneficial components of human milk are completely destroyed during heat processing of milk. This is untrue. Many components are decreased during processing, and a few are destroyed totally, but the bioactivity of processed human milk still exceeds that of formula which contains no immune properties at all and many other components that are not even kingdom- or phylum-specific, let alone species-specific! In a study conducted jointly by the FDA and the CDC in 1990, banked donor milk was processed and analyzed for content.[15] The goal of the study was threefold: (1) to validate results of much older studies using newer analytical techniques, (2) to explore whether large amounts of bacteria could be destroyed routinely at a lower temperature; and, (3) to determine whether heating banked milk at a lower temperature would be beneficial.

Eitenmiller used the HMBANA guidelines for processing milk, duplicating the type of equipment used and the volumes processed. The milk was inoculated with 1 million colony-forming units (10^6 CFU/ml) of each marker bacteria, both *S. aureus and E. coli.* Milk was treated at either 56° C or 62.5° C. for thirty minutes. The results of Eitenmiller's study closely parallel early studies in the approximate amounts of components remaining after heat treatment and are shown in Table 12.1. All the marker bacteria are destroyed at both temperatures. The nutritional properties of the milk are most stable. Significant amounts of immune components also remain, with the lower temperatures resulting in greater preservation of components.

The exception to this are some of the enzymes inherent in human milk. These enzymes are most beneficial to preterm infants who lack mature enzyme systems of their own for digestion. The enzymes in human milk complement those of the infant's gastrointestinal tract. One of the most important, bile salt-stimulated lipase (or bile salt-dependent lipase), begins to decrease even as milk is warmed to just slightly above body temperature. Hamosh and colleagues estimate as much as 15–20 percent is gone when milk reaches 38° C (100.4° F) and is completely gone when milk reaches 56° C.[16] The implications for banked donor milk are that utilization of nutrients may be slightly less efficient in the preterm infant when banked donor milk is compared with the infant's

TABLE 12.1   Effects of Heat on Milk Composition[17]

Component	56 ° C	62.5 ° C
Bacteria:		
S. aureus & E. coli	100% killed	100% killed
Lactoferrin	72% left	22% left
IgA	84% left	51% left
Folic Acid	72% left	57% left
Lysozyme	132% left	100% left
Phosphatase	23% left	1.4% left

mother's own milk that has not been processed. Other enzymes, such as amylase, are more impervious to heat.

Debates about the adequacy of banked donor milk for the preterm infant are ongoing. Because the milk is collected primarily from women who are nursing older term infants and pooled, is it age-appropriate for a preterm infant? Milk banks do make an effort to segregate donor milk from preterm mothers (defined as the first four weeks of lactation in a mother delivering an infant younger than thirty-seven weeks' gestation) because of its special composition and will preferentially provide that milk to premature recipients. However, term milk has been used in the past with no deleterious effects. Banked donor milk can be fortified with the additional calcium and phosphorus required for preterm bone mineralization, and other fortifiers can also be added as needed by the infant, just the way fortification of a mother's own milk would be done.

One should remember, however, that *banked donor milk is the only transplanted tissue that retains its functional properties and bioactivity after heat treatment.*

Accessibility of Banked Donor Milk

Donor milk banking is an equation that is not always very balanced. Ideally, supply meets demand. Because banked donor milk is a prescription item, the physician or other prescriber is at the heart of the accessibility issue. Many physicians have never heard of donor milk banks or are unaware of the precautions that have been put in place to protect the recipient population from disease transmission. Some continue the distrust of wet nurses that was prevalent at the end of the nineteenth and beginning of the twentieth centuries.[18]

Fees associated with donor milk banking also affect accessibility of banked donor milk. Donor milk banks in the United States charge a processing fee for the milk, which averaged $2.75 per ounce in 2001. The recipient family is paying for a portion of the screening costs and costs of processing the milk to ensure a safe product. While the costs per ounce for donor screening decrease as the donor gives more and more milk, economies of scale are not always possible during processing as each ounce must be treated the same way. Processing is labor-intensive, bacteriological testing is costly, and batch loads are small. The processing fee of $2.75 per ounce does not begin to meet the actual costs of providing a safe product, nor has the price been raised for approximately fifteen years, possibly making banked donor milk the "sleeper" bargain of the year. Milk banks do not make money, and many do not even break even, with the hosting hospital covering the deficit as a community service and/or supplying many in-kind costs.

One would like to think that banked donor milk is covered by insurance; after all, it is a prescription. This is not the case, however. Many insurers will not pay for special foods, therefore, they will not cover banked donor milk because it is classified as a food. Another argument is that it is not listed in the "formulary." Getting insurance coverage from third-party payers is more difficult than getting coverage from Medicaid, although coverage by the latter is based on individual state policy, not federal policy. However, no recipient is denied access to donor milk for inability to pay. In 1996 the Denver Mothers' Milk Bank wrote off approximately $80,000 in uncollectible processing fees.[19]

Pitfalls of Informal Sharing

Strong recommendations exist against the informal sharing of human milk. Even with serological screening, with informal sharing the additional safety of heat treatment is missing. Some women do not know they are at risk for transmissible diseases; a partner's extracurricular sexual behavior may be extremely well hidden and unknown to the potential donor, or she may be unwilling to acknowledge that she is at risk and self-exclude. Yet many mothers know that human milk is the best thing for their infants. They may feel forced to go to great extremes to acquire human milk if they cannot access the formal milk banking system. In the age of the Internet and World Wide Web, this is particularly worrisome as individuals with good intentions and little understanding of the issues try and set up web sites where potential donors and potential recipient families can register and connect themselves together with no screening precautions, no bacteriological quality control, and no pasteurization. The risk of disease transmission is increased dramatically, and liability abounds for both the donor and the person maintaining the web site who is condoning this informal sharing.

Additionally, there is no regulation about whether a supplier of milk can receive payment for her milk in this uncontrolled system. For some there would be the temptation to increase their income by padding their milk supply, either through the addition of cow's milk or water. In the case of the infant allergic to cow's milk protein, this could be a lethal arrangement.

If informal sharing arrangements become more commonplace, the damage to milk banking services in general could be extreme, and all donated milk would be tarnished by association.[20]

Clinical Uses of Banked Donor Milk

The need for donor milk may be either a nutritional need, a medicinal or therapeutic need, or a need for prevention (= health protection).[21] For the fragile infant, all three purposes may be accomplished with the clinical use of banked donor milk. For example, the preterm infant receives nutrition while the dose of donor milk reduces the risk of contracting necrotizing enterocolitis. Additionally, the infant is being supplied therapeutic doses of immunoglobulins to complement its immature immune system as well as therapeutic doses of growth factors to support growth and maturation of tissues and organs in an extrauterine environment. Table 12.2 supports the benefits of feeding human milk to preterm babies. For the adult recipient, clinical use is much more apt to be medicinal or therapeutic only (e.g., providing IgA to an IgA-deficient patient), rather than preventive or nutritional.

Frequently there may be more than one problem in a very sick infant, making diagnosis and proper treatment of the problem difficult. In these cases a short-term, temporary use of donor milk may buy the practitioner some time to make an accurate diagnosis without doing further harm to the infant. With the exception of the rare genetic disorder of galactosemia (incidence about 1:50,000 births), for which any milk containing lactose is contraindicated, banked donor milk will do no harm.[22] The clinical uses of banked donor milk are well described.[23]

Around the world, countries with donor milk banking services use banked donor milk nearly exclusively for preterm infants. An infant who does not have access to his or her own mother's milk will be fed donor milk. This is not the case in the United States, where milk banks have managed to remain operational by treating medical conditions in sick infants, children, and the occasional adult. In the 1970s at the height of donor milk banking in the U.S., approximately 90 percent of the milk dispensed went to preterm infants. Today only about 40 percent of the volume goes to preterm infants.[24] The advent of preterm

TABLE 12.2   Growth in Preterm Infants Fed Different Types of Feedings[25]

Goal	Group A Mom's Milk (n = 11)	Group B Donor milk* (n = 12)	Group C Preterm Formula (n = 21)
Regain birth weight	22 days	18 days	19 days
Achieve 2,000 grams	55 days	54 days	49 days

*Donor milk collected only in first 8 days of lactation, e.g. colostrum and transitional milk.

formulas and a renewed emphasis on using the mother's own milk have reduced the use of donor milk in the NICU, although this is not necessarily the desired outcome for either milk banks or preterm infants who do not have access to their mother's own milk.[26]

Cost effectiveness can be demonstrated through the use of donor milk, despite the expense of the processing fee. Several cases of clinical use in infants with accompanying cost savings have been presented in a previous publication.[27] These cases range from savings of several thousand dollars to hundreds of thousands of dollars and cover cases of infants as well as adults. What is notable with premature infants, however, is that the cost of the donor milk is inconsequential compared to the savings in earlier discharge and lack of added costs due to NEC, sepsis, or other complications. Using direct hospital costs, Wight has calculated that if donor milk is as effective in preventing NEC and sepsis and shortening hospital stays for preterm infants, for every $1 spent on donor milk the NICU saves between $11 and $37 in NICU costs.[28] Arnold has used two other models, the charge model and the costs to an individual state, to calculate potential savings from NEC prevention alone.[29]

Perhaps the most common reason for using banked donor milk in the United States is formula "intolerance," or severe allergy to human milk substitutes. Case after case is seen by milk banks where multiple formulas have been tried on an infant with no change in the infant's symptoms. In many such cases, the introduction of donor milk resolves the symptoms within twenty-four hours.

Perhaps the most famous case of formula intolerance is the case of Lacie, who at age twenty still requires a substantial amount of human milk in her diet and probably will continue to do so for her entire life.[30] Additional instances of clinical uses of donor milk have been published.[31] One of the largest criticisms that can be leveled at the use of banked donor milk is that there is very little research which proves its efficacy. What we have in large part is a body of anecdotal knowledge, a record of the diagnoses (but not the outcomes) for which milk was prescribed from various milk banks, and a few published case histories. For rare conditions, case control studies would be a solution, but what is needed is randomized prospective trials.

International Perspective

A few other countries have donor milk banking services. While officials of the World Health Organization privately acknowledge the need for donor milk in many settings, statements favoring donor milk banking services or the use of milk from another woman through wet nursing has become mired in HIV politics, with government officials who know little about breastfeeding and child survival making decisions based on fear and lack of knowledge. The World Health Organization keeps no list of nations with milk banking services, and although it has funded conferences in the past on milk banking, it has not done so since HIV became an issue. According to some sources, UNICEF has also spent money on donor milk banking equipment in Latin American countries, but the status of milk banking in these places is unknown to this author. Obviously, it is easier to develop milk banking services in countries where infrastructures are reliable.

Milk banking services in Europe are the best known. Donor milk banking originated there in the early 1900s, simultaneously with and independent of its creation in the United States. Milk banking standards are incorporated into the body of public health laws and regulations, and the clinical use of donor milk is covered under national health services. Pediatric societies have relatively recent statements that support the use of banked donor milk. An example from the Nutrition Committee of the German Pediatric Society follows:

> Donor milk is needed as an important option for the care and treatment of premature and sick newborns and babies. Its use in pediatrics has a primarily preventive and therapeutic character, particularly with immature newborns and in cases of serious intestinal illness in infancy, such as NEC, Morbus Hirschprung, intractable diarrhea and cow's milk protein allergy.[32]

Supply, however, limits many of these countries to primarily serving preterm infants, with very few sick infants receiving donor milk. Discussions of different international milk banking practices may be found in a variety of publications.[33]

Perhaps the most elaborate donor milk banking system is in Brazil where donor milk banking services are incorporated into the national breastfeeding promotion campaign. With more than 150 milk banks, Brazil is the record-holder for sheer numbers of milk banks. These milk banks are an integral part of the health care system. There is one milk bank which acts as a reference milk bank, establishing standards for milk banks, conducting research on processing and composition and clinical uses, and undertaking large education programs including training of all hospital staff under the Baby-Friendly Hospital Initiative.[34]

In contrast, the U.S. donor milk banking community operates without federal support in terms of either legislation or policy statements. Donor milk banks are not regulated except in the states of California and New York where they must be licensed tissue banks operating under state health regulations. Nor has the American Academy of Pediatrics taken any stand on donor milk banking in the form of a policy statement since 1980 (pre-HIV) although there are occasional updates about donor milk banking in the *AAP Red Book on Infectious Diseases,* the *Pediatric Nutrition Handbook,* and *Guidelines for Perinatal Care,* all of which act as policy statements.[35] The Canadian Pediatric Society, on the other hand, has issued a very negative and uneducated statement about donor milk banking which misinterprets the research literature and flagrantly ignores established guidelines.[36] This is in contrast to the German statement above and the situation in Britain where the Nutrition Committee of the British Pediatric Society actually helped create the guidelines for donor milk banking with milk bank coordinators and published them as well.[37]

Needs for the Future

Internationally, the World Health Organization is the ideal organization to take the lead and put donor milk banking into GOBI. Not only is donor milk a promoter of growth in infants at risk, it is oral rehydration with medicinal properties, it is breast milk feeding if not breastfeeding, and it is immunization. Breastfeeding needs to be removed from the political HIV arena, especially in developed countries where adequate screening techniques and processing of donated milk can be easily done.

In the United States, milk banking needs to be brought into the mainstream. The basic issues are to improve access to donor milk and to improve its quality.

- The Public Health Service, in the body of the CDC and working with the FDA and the U.S. Department of Agriculture, should establish policies favoring the use of donor milk. Regulation of milk banks would help establish credibility with prescribers. (*access, quality*)
- The CDC should work with the American Academy of Pediatrics (AAP) and other organizations to develop a positive policy statement about donor milk banking, its benefits and its clinical uses, and to establish research priorities. (*access, quality*)
- Research priorities should be funded by NIH with funds that are in addition to funding already in place for basic research on human milk composition and growth. Researchers should be urged to include donor milk arms in feeding studies. (*quality*)
- Research on new technologies for processing human milk while protecting its safety and causing the least damage to milk components should be conducted. Processing should be taken to a larger, more efficient scale, and techniques from other countries should be investigated and incorporated into U.S. methodologies. Grants to milk banks for new equipment should be made available. (*quality, access*)

- Labeling donor milk should be improved, and further screening tests should be incorporated (drug screens of milk itself, nutrient labels, better segregation of lactational stages). (*quality*)
- The supply of donor milk should be made more readily available so that it is just as easy to "pull off the shelf" as formula. (*access*)
- Insurance companies should be educated that donor milk is not just a "food" and that there are cost savings to be seen with its use so that they will cover the cost of donor milk to the recipient. (*access*)
- In the absence of uniform third-party coverage for donor milk, government health care programs such as Medicare, Medicaid, and WIC should cover donor milk. (*access*)
- A better network of milk banking services should be set up nationwide so that donors and recipients in all states can be easily served. Regionalization is the most cost-effective method of offering donor milk banking services. However, a few milk banks cannot be expected to handle an increased demand for milk, as they are close to being overextended now. (*access*)
- The AAP Breastfeeding Work Group should take the initiative to come up with a new donor milk banking statement that addresses the issues of disease transmission and the hazards of informal sharing of milk, and then supply its members with information on accessing banked donor milk safely. The imperative is even greater now with access to the Internet and people sharing and selling all sorts of tissues and organs over the Internet. (*access, quality*)
- Breastfeeding education should become an integral and required part of the education that all doctors, nurses, and dietitians must have, no matter what the specialty of the health professional will be in the end. Only when all health professionals understand the importance of human milk will progress be made in maternal and child health. It is appalling that books relating to the feeding of "at-risk" infants and toddlers mention breastfeeding only in passing and never mention banked donor milk as an option.[38] Additionally, without basic knowledge of human milk composition, there will be a general lack of understanding and willingness to use donor milk in innovative therapies, such as adjunct cancer therapy. (*access*)
- Funding should be made available to market donor milk as an acceptable alternative to formula in the absence of mother's own milk. (*access*)
- Use of banked donor milk should be incorporated into the assessment for a Baby-Friendly Hospital. (*access*)

Summary

The clinical use of donor milk is critical to the survival of many infants and children. Without accurate knowledge about the process of donor milk banking, the benefits of donor milk, and its potential clinical uses, prescribers will continue to be unaware of its accessibility in the United States and will continue to have negative and incorrect impressions of banked donor milk. In this regard, education of health care providers and appropriate marketing of banked donor milk is essential to the growth of these services and improved access to all potential recipients, whether or not they are infants. Development of a cohesive federal policy on breastfeeding and the use of human milk based on the United States Breastfeeding Committee's Strategic Plan will provide a basis for ensuring access to lactation care and services, including access to donor milk for those infants without access to their own mother's milk. Only then will the issues outlined in this chapter be addressed.

References and Notes

1. World Health Organization/United Nations Children's Fund. 1980. Meeting on infant and young child feeding. *J. Nurse Midwif.* 25: 31–38.
2. World Health Organization/United Nations Children's Fund. 1992. Consensus statement from the WHO/UNICEF consultation on HIV transmission and breast-feeding, Geneva, April 30-May 1.
3. Food and Drug Administration, Office of Orphan Product Development. 1988. Clinical studies of safety and effectiveness of orphan products: Availability of grants; requests for applications. Federal Register, 53: 44951.
4. Arnold, L. D. W. 1996. *The Role of Donor Milk in the Reduction of Infant Mortality and Morbidity: A Child Survival Issue.* Health Education Associates: Sandwich, MA.
   Arnold, L. D. W., and L. L. Borman. 1996. What are the characteristics of the ideal human milk donor? *J. Hum. Lact.* 12: 143.
5. Human Milk Banking Association of North America. 2000. *Guidelines for the Establishment and Operation of a Donor Human Milk Bank.* Tully, M. R., ed. Raleigh, NC.
6. For an overview of donor milk banking operations see: Arnold, L. D. W. 1997. Donor milk banking in the United States: The state of the art. *ABM News and Views* 3(4): 5, 7.
   Arnold, L. D. W. 1997. How North American donor milk banks operate: Results of a survey, Part 1. *J. Hum. Lact.* 13(2): 159.
   Arnold, L. D. W. 1997. How North American donor milk banks operate: Results of a survey, Part 2. *J. Hum. Lact.* 13(3): 243.

Langerak, E. R., and L. D. W. Arnold. 1991. The Mothers' Milk Bank of Wilmington, Delaware: History and highlights. *J. Hum. Lact.* 7: 197.

7. United States Department of Health and Human Services, Public Health Service. 1994. Guidelines for Preventing Transmission of Human Immunodeficiency Virus Through Transplantation of Human Tissue and Organs. *MMWR* Vol. 43, No. RR-8, May 20.

8. Arnold, L. D. W. 2001. Trends in donor milk banking in the United States. In Newburg D, ed. *Bioactive Substances in Human Milk.* New York: Plenum Press. 509.

9. Eglin, R. P., and A. R. Wilkinson. 1987. HIV infection and pasteurisation of breast milk. *Lancet* 1: 1093.
Orloff, S. L. et al. 1993. Inactivation of human immunodeficiency virus type I in human milk: Effects of intrinsic factors in human milk and of pasteurization. *J. Hum. Lact.* 9: 13.

10. Arnold, L. D. W. 1998. How to order banked donor milk in the United States: What the health care provider needs to know. *J. Hum. Lact.* 14(1): 65.

11. Arnold, L. D. W. 1996. Possibilities for donor milk use in adult clinical settings—A largely unexplored area. *J. Hum. Lact.* 12: 56.
Arnold, L. D. W. 1998. Cost savings through the use of donor milk: Case histories. *J. Hum. Lact.* 14(3): 255.
Wiggins, P. K., and L. D. W. Arnold. 1998. Clinical case history: Donor milk use for severe gastroesophageal reflux in an adult. *J. Hum. Lact.* 14(2): 157.

12. Arnold, L. D. W., and E. Larson. 1993. Immunologic benefits of breast milk in relation to human milk banking. *Amer. J. Infec. Control* 21: 235.

13. Arnold, L. D. W. 1998. Cost savings through the use of donor milk: Case histories.
Merhav, H. J. et al. 1995. Treatment of IgA deficiency in liver transplant recipients with human breast milk. *Transpl. Int.* 8: 327.

14. Arnold, L. D. W. 1996. *The Role of Donor Milk in the Reduction of Infant Mortality and Morbidity: A Child Survival Issue.* Health Education Associates: Sandwich MA, 13, 27–28.

15. Eitenmiller, R. 1990. An overview of human milk pasteurization. Presentation at the annual meeting of the Human Milk Banking Association of North America, Inc. Lexington, KY, October 15.

16. Hamosh, M. et al. 1997. Digestive enzymes in human milk: Stability at suboptimal storage temperatures. *J. Pediatr. Gastroent. Nutr.* 24: 38.

17. Eitenmiller, R. 1990.

18. Golden, J. 1996. *A Social History of Wet Nursing in America: From Breast to Bottle.* Cambridge University Press: New York.

19. Borman, L. L., personal communication.

20. Arnold, L. D. W. 1994. Informal sharing of human milk: Not-so-hypothetical questions, concrete answers. *J. Hum. Lact.* 10: 43.

21. Arnold, L. D. W. 1999. Donor human milk banking: More than nutrition. Chapter 24 in Riordan, J., and K. G. Auerbach, eds. *Breastfeeding and Human Lactation,* 2nd edition. Sudbury, MA: Jones and Bartlett Publishers. 775.

Arnold, L. D. W. 1999. Use of banked donor milk in the United States. *Building Block for Life* (Newsletter of the Pediatric Nutrition Practice Group of Amer. Diet. Assoc.) 23(1): 1, 3–6, Winter.

22. Thoene, J. G., ed. 1995. *Physicians' Guide to Rare Diseases,* 2nd edition. Montvale, NJ: Dowden Publishing Co., Inc. 194.

23. Arnold, L. D. W. 1990. Clinical uses of donor milk. *J. Human Lact.* 6: 132.

    Arnold, L. D. W. 1999. Donor human milk banking: More than nutrition.

    Arnold, L. D. W. 1999. Use of banked donor milk in the United States.

    Asquith, M., et al. 1987. Clinical uses, collection, and banking of human milk. *Clins. Perinatol.* 14: 173.

24. Arnold, L. D. W. 1997. How North American donor milk banks operate: Results of a survey, Part 2.

25. Zachou, T. 1996. Growth in preterm infants fed different types of feedings. Oral presentation at the annual meeting of the Human Milk Banking Association of North America, Inc., Raleigh, NC, March 1.

26. Arnold, L. D. W. 1993. Human milk for premature infants: An important health issue. *J. Hum. Lact.* 9: 116.

    Arnold, L. D. W. 1994. Donor human milk for premature infants: The famous case of the Dionne quintuplets. *J. Hum. Lact.* 10: 271.

27. Arnold, L. D. W. 1998. Cost savings through the use of donor milk: Case histories.

28. Wight, N. E. 2001. Donor human milk for preterm infants. *J. Perinatol.* 21: 249.

29. Arnold, L. D. W. 2002. The cost effectiveness of using banked donor milk in the neonatal intensive care unit: Prevention of necrotizing enterocolitis. *J. Hum. Lact.* 18: in press.

30. Arnold, L. D. W. 1995. Use of donor milk in the treatment of metabolic disorders: Glycolytic pathway defects. *J. Hum. Lact.* 11: 51.

31. Anderson, A., and L. D. W. Arnold. 1993. Use of donor breastmilk in the nutrition management of chronic renal failure: Three case histories. *J. Hum. Lact.* 9: 263.

    Arnold, L. D. W. 1995. Use of donor milk in the management of failure to thrive: Case histories. *J. Hum. Lact.* 11: 137.

    Rangecroft, L. et al. 1978. A comparison of the feeding of the postoperative newborn with banked breast-milk or cow's-milk feeds. *J. Pediatr. Surg.* 13: 11.

    Riddell, D. 1989. Use of banked human milk for feeding infants with abdominal wall defects. Presentation at the annual meeting of the Human Milk Banking Association of North America, Inc., Vancouver, BC, Canada, October 15.

    Tully, M. R. 1990. Banked human milk in the treatment of IgA deficiency and allergy symptoms. *J. Hum. Lact.* 6: 75.

32. As translated in Springer, S. 1997. Human milk banking in Germany. *J. Hum. Lact.* 13: 65.

33. Arnold, L. D. W. 1994. The lactariums of France: Part 1. The Lactarium Docteur Raymond Fourcade in Marmande. *J. Hum. Lact.* 10: 125.

Arnold, L. D. W. 1996. Donor milk banking in China: The ultimate step in becoming Baby Friendly. *J. Hum. Lact.,* 12: 319.

Arnold, L. D. W. 1999. Donor milk banking in Scandinavia. *J. Hum. Lact.* 15: 55.

Arnold, L. D. W., and M. Courdent. 1994. The lactariums of France, Part 2: How association milk banks operate. *J. Hum. Lact.* 10: 195.

Balmer, S. E. 1995. Donor milk banking and guidelines in Britain. *J. Hum. Lact.* 1: 229.

Fernandez, A. et al. 1993. The establishment of a human milk bank in India. *J. Hum. Lact.* 9: 189.

Penc, B. 1996. Organization and activity of a human milk bank in Poland. *J. Hum. Lact.* 12: 243.

Springer, S. 1997. Human milk banking in Germany.

34. Gutierrez, D., and J. A. G. Almeida. 1998. Human milk banks in Brazil. *J. Hum. Lact.* 14: 333.

35. American Academy of Pediatrics, Committee on Nutrition. 1980. Human milk banking. *Pediatrics,* 65: 854.

American Academy of Pediatrics, Committee on Infectious Diseases. 1997. *1997 Red Book,* 24th edition. AAP: Elk Grove Village, IL, 76.

American Academy of Pediatrics, Committee on Nutrition. 1998. *Pediatric Nutrition Handbook,* 4th edition. AAP: Elk Grove Village, IL, 70.

American Academy of Pediatrics and the American College of Obstetricians and Gynecologists. 1997. *Guidelines for Perinatal Care,* 4th edition. AAP/ACOG: Elk Grove Village, IL, 288.

36. Canadian Paediatric Society, Nutrition Committee. 1995. Human milk banking and storage. Statement No. 95-03. CPS: Toronto.

The Canadian statement has been nullified recently, but this has not been widely publicized. A new statement more supportive of donor milk banking is in the process of being developed. Janice Wensley, personal communication, June 2001.

37. Balmer, S. E. 1995. Donor milk banking and guidelines in Britain. Springer, S. 1997.

38. Cox, J. H., ed. 1997. *Nutrition Manual for At-Risk Infants and Toddlers.* Precept Press: Chicago.

CONCLUSION

Four themes, five synergies, and two mandates emerged from our process of crystallization. These themes, synergies, and mandates were also reflected in Karin's, Cindy's, and Lois's contributions to the United States Breastfeeding Committee's Strategic Plan, *Protecting, Promoting and Supporting Breastfeeding in the United States: A National Agenda and the Health and Human Services Blueprint for Action on Breastfeeding* that was being developed in tandem with this volume. It is our belief that they are the guideposts for reclaiming breastfeeding.

The four themes are

1. **The significance of breastfeeding promotion, protection, and support in the U.S. health care system, in particular, and in social policy, in general.** Well-done research and economic analysis continues to indicate that breastfeeding, especially exclusive breastfeeding for the first six months and continuing through the first year and beyond, would save a minimum of $3.6 billion a year if increased from current levels to those recommended by the Surgeon General.[1]

2. **The ongoing need for routine collection of data regarding breastfeeding incidence, duration, exclusivity, and data related to the quality of care and practice outcomes for breastfeeding support and services.** This theme has been recognized as vital by the federal governmental, which is now collecting nationwide data. Community and practice data is needed to provide quality services on the local level, especially to reduce disparity of care and to identify opportunities to offer cooperative services and seamless care.

3. **The importance of evidence-based practices related to breastfeeding support and services within the health care system, including the implementation of the Baby-Friendly**

Hospital Initiative. Research is needed relating to practice and service delivery in order to design evidence-based management strategies. Practice guidelines of the WHO/UNICEF Baby-Friendly Hospital Initiative should be designed for out-of-hospital lactation management practice. Implementation of the BFHI should be extended beyond the approximate 1 percent of United States hospitals participating in 2001.

4. **The value and need for preservice training and continuing education related to breastfeeding support and service in the health care system.** Every published research study indicates that physicians, nurses, and other health care providers receive less than adequate preservice training related to breastfeeding management. Substantial improvement is essential to reclaiming breastfeeding in the United States.

The five synergies[2] are

1. **Improving breastfeeding outcomes by coordinating lactation support and services.** This synergy would ensure seamless support for mothers and babies. Prenatal care, hospital care, and post-partum care would be continuous and not contradictory. Mothers and babies would receive coordinated services even if the services were provided at different sites. Ideally, "one-stop" mother-baby centers would be developed in neighborhoods, and lactation support and services would be integrated into existing sites.

    Barros reported the impact of community lactation centers in a study of demographically matched neighborhoods in Brazil.[3] After adjusting for confounders, the breastfeeding rate at four months was 43 percent (versus only 18 percent in the matched neighborhood without a lactation center), and at six months the breastfeeding rate was 15 percent (versus 6 percent in the matched neighborhood without a lactation center). Weight for age was also significantly better in those infants breastfed in the neighborhood with the lactation center. This study has not been replicated in the United States.

2. **Improving access to care by establishing frameworks to pay for lactation support services.** This synergy encourages the provision of skilled breastfeeding support in every community along with community referral networks for breastfeeding support and services. Also included in this synergy would be the elimination of disparity in breastfeeding rates among populations of women. Third-party payers should pay for lactation support and services in the same manner that other health promoting services are funded.

3. **Improving the quality and cost-effectiveness of breastfeeding care and services by applying a population perspective to practice.** This synergy includes using population information and strategies to enhance clinical decision making and to "funnel" patients to medical care. In order to implement this synergy for breastfeeding effectively, outcomes and incidence data should be collected in the community and reported to individual medical practitioners. Up to this point breastfeeding promotion and support has not been a subject of medical accountability.

4. **Using the clinical practice of providing lactation support to identify and address community health problems.** This synergy encourages the use of clinical encounters related to breastfeeding to build a communitywide database as well as to identify and address underlying causes of breastfeeding problems. This synergy would involve the identification of features of mothers who use breastfeeding support services as well as the reasons for their seeking those services. Encounters with the health care system would be used to identify why women choose to breastfeed or not and the breastfeeding issues the women identify as current, past, or future problems.

5. **Shaping the future by collaborating around breastfeeding policy, training and research.** This synergy promotes collaboration in order to develop and implement evidence-based influence health system policies and procedures and to engage in cross-sectoral education and training and conduct cross-sectoral research.

The two mandates are

1. **Improve the quality of care and services related to breastfeeding and human lactation.**
2. **Identify and remove barriers to breastfeeding and lactation care services.**

References

1. Weimer, J. 2001. The Economic Benefits of Breastfeeding: A Review and Analysis. Food and Rural Economics Division, Economic Research Service, United States Department of Agriculture. Food Assistance and Nutrition Research Report No. 13.
2. The synergies were adapted from those suggested for public health and medicine in Lasker, R. D., 1997. *Medicine and Public Health: The Power of Collaboration.* New York: The New York Academy of Medicine, 41.
3. Barros, B. 1995f. The impact of lactation centers on breastfeeding rates. *Acta. Paediatrica* 84: 1221.

INNOCENTI DECLARATION

Innocenti Declaration

On the Protection, Promotion and Support of Breastfeeding. 1 August, 1990, Florence, Italy

Recognising that

Breastfeeding is a unique process that:

- Provides ideal nutrition for infants and contributes to their healthy growth and development
- Reduces incidence and severity of infectious diseases, thereby lowering infant morbidity and mortality
- Contributes to women's health by reducing the risk of breast and ovarian cancer, and by increasing the spacing between pregnancies
- Provides social and economic benefits to the family and the nation
- Provides most women with a sense of satisfaction when successfully carried out

and that Recent Research has found that:

- these benefits increase with increased exclusiveness[1] of breastfeeding during the first six months of life, and thereafter with increased duration of breastfeeding with complementary foods, and
- programme intervention can result in positive changes in breastfeeding behaviour

We Therefore Declare that:

As a global goal for optimal maternal and child health and nutrition, all women should be enabled to practise exclusive breastfeeding and all infants should be fed exclusively on breast milk from birth to 4–6 months of age. Thereafter, children should continue to be breastfed, while receiving appropriate and adequate complementary foods, for up to two years of age or beyond. This child-feeding ideal is to be achieved by creating an appropriate environment of awareness and support so that women can breastfeed in this manner.

Attainment of this goal requires, in many countries, the reinforcement of a "breastfeeding culture" and its vigorous defence against incursions of a "bottle-feeding culture." This requires commitment and advocacy for social mobilization, utilizing to the full the prestige and authority of acknowledged leaders of society in all walks of life.

Efforts should be made to increase women's confidence in their ability to breastfeed. Such empowerment involves the removal of constraints and influences that manipulate perceptions and behaviour towards breastfeeding, often by subtle and indirect means. This requires sensitivity, continued vigilance, and a responsive and comprehensive communications strategy involving all media and addressed to all levels of society. Furthermore, obstacles to breastfeeding within the health system, the workplace and the community must be eliminated.

Measures should be taken to ensure that women are adequately nourished for their optimal health and that of their families. Furthermore, ensuring that all women also have access to family planning information and services allows them to sustain breastfeeding and avoid shortened birth intervals that may compromise their health and nutritional status, and that of their children.

All governments should develop national breastfeeding policies and set appropriate national targets for the 1990s. They should establish a national system for monitoring the attainment of their targets, and they should develop indicators such as the prevalence of exclusively breastfed infants at discharge from maternity services, and the prevalence of exclusively breastfed infants at four months of age.

National authorities are further urged to integrate their breastfeeding policies into their overall health and development policies. In so doing they should reinforce all actions that protect, promote and support breastfeeding within complementary programmes such as prenatal and perinatal care, nutrition, family planning services, and prevention and treatment of common maternal and childhood diseases. All healthcare staff should be trained in the skills necessary to implement these breastfeeding policies.

Operational Targets

All governments by the year 1995 should have:

- Appointed a national breastfeeding coordinator of appropriate authority, and established a multisectoral national breastfeeding committee composed of representatives from relevant government departments, non-governmental organizations, and health professional associations
- Ensured that every facility providing maternity services fully practises all ten of the Ten Steps to Successful Breastfeeding set out in the joint WHO/UNICEF statement "Protecting, promoting and supporting breastfeeding: the special role of maternity services."[2]
- Taken action to give effect to the principles and aim of all Articles of the International Code of Marketing of Breast-Milk Substitutes and subsequent relevant World Health Assembly resolutions in their entirety; and
- Enacted imaginative legislation protecting the breastfeeding rights of working women and established means for its enforcement.

We also call upon international organizations to:

- Draw up action strategies for protecting, promoting and supporting breastfeeding, including global monitoring and evaluation of their strategies.
- Support national situation analyses and surveys and the development of national goals and targets for action; and
- Encourage and support national authorities in planning, implementing, monitoring and evaluating their breastfeeding policies

References

1. Exclusive breastfeeding means that no other drink or food is given to the infant; the infant should feed frequently and for unrestricted periods.
2. World Health Organization, Geneva, 1989.

The Innocenti Declaration was produced and adopted by participants at the WHO/UNICEF policymakers' meeting on "Breastfeeding in the 1990s: A Global Initiative, co-sponsored by the United States Agency for International Development (A.I.D.) and the Swedish International Development Authority (SIDA), held at the Spedale degli Innocenti," Florence, Italy, on 30 July–1 August 1990. The Declaration reflects the content of the original background document for the meeting and the views expressed in group and plenary sessions.

INTERNATIONAL CODE OF MARKETING OF BREAST MILK SUBSTITUTES

Summary

No advertising of infant formula, pacifiers or feeding bottles to the public.

No free samples to mothers.

No promotion of infant feeding products (e.g., by notepads, booklets, posters, displays) in health care facilities.

No company mothercraft nurses to advise mothers.

No gifts of personal samples to health workers.

No words or pictures idealizing artificial feeding, including pictures of infants, on the labels of the products.

Information to health workers should be scientific and factual.

All information on artificial infant feeding, including the labels, should explain the benefits of breastfeeding, *and* the costs and hazards associated with artificial feeding.

Unsuitable products, such as sweetened condensed milk and evaporated milk, should not be promoted for babies.

All products should be of a high quality and take account of the climatic and storage conditions of the country where they are used.

World Health Organization, 1985.

APPENDIX C

OVERVIEW OF GOALS AND OBJECTIVES OF THE U.S. NATIONAL AGENDA

Goal I: Assure access to comprehensive, current, and culturally appropriate lactation care and services for all women, children, and families.

Objective IA	Identify and disseminate evidence-based best practices and polices throughout the health care system.
Objective IB	Educate all health care providers and payers regarding appropriate breastfeeding and lactation support.
Objective IC	Ensure that all women have access to appropriate breastfeeding support within the family and/or community.
Objective ID	Ensure the routine collection and coordination of breastfeeding data by federal, state, and local government and other organizations, and foster additional breastfeeding research.

United States Breastfeeding Committee. 2001. Breastfeeding in the United States: A National Agenda. Rockville, MD: United States Department of Health and Human Services, Health Resources and Services Administration, Maternal and Child Health Bureau.

Goal II: Ensure that breastfeeding is recognized as the normal and preferred method of feeding infants and young children.

Objective IIA   Develop a positive and desirable image of breast-feeding for the American public.

Objective IIB   Reduce the barriers to breastfeeding posed by the marketing of breast milk substitutes.

Goal III: Ensure that all Federal, State, and local laws relating to child welfare and family law recognize and support the importance and practice of breastfeeding.

Objective IIIA   Ensure that all lawmakers and government officials at Federal, State, and local levels are aware of the importance of protecting, promoting, and supporting breastfeeding.

Goal IV: Increase protection, promotion, and support for breastfeeding mothers in the work force.

Objective IVA   The rights of women in the workplace will be recognized in public and private sectors.

Objective IVB   Ensure that all mothers are able to seamlessly integrate breastfeeding and employment.

BLUEPRINT FOR ACTION ON BREASTFEEDING

Infants should be exclusively breastfed during the first 4 to 6 months of life, preferably for a full 6 months. Ideally, breastfeeding should continue through the first year of life. This Blueprint for Action reaffirms the scientific evidence that breastfeeding is the best method for feeding most newborns, and that breastfeeding is beneficial to the infant's and the mother's health. Achieving an increase in the proportion of mothers who breastfeed their babies will require the collaboration of Federal agencies, State and local governments, communities, health professional organizations, advocacy groups, multidisciplinary scientists, industry, health insurers, and the American people. This Blueprint for Action invites all interested stakeholders to forge partnerships for the promotion of breastfeeding. It is also designed to attract broad-based family, community, professional, corporate, and philanthropic participation in order to better focus the public's attention and to motivate actions at the individual and community levels.

Moreover, this Blueprint for Action is directed toward all women and cuts across all racial and ethnic populations, socio-economic classes, educational groups, and employment arrangements. It concentrates energy in key breastfeeding promotion domains and denotes

United States Department of Health and Human Services. 2000. *HHS Blueprint for Action on Breastfeeding.* Washington, DC: Office on Women's Health.

responsibility for a definitive course of action by the various stakeholders to achieve a greater proportion of breastfeeding mothers in
American society.

To achieve the Healthy People 2010 Breastfeeding Objectives for the
Nation, the Blueprint for Action recommends that the following steps
be taken by the health care system, the workplace, the family, and the
community, and identifies several areas of research.

Health Care System

- Train health care professionals who provide maternal and child
  care on the basics of lactation, breastfeeding counseling, and
  lactation management during coursework, clinical and in-service
  training, and continuing education.
- Ensure that breastfeeding mothers have access to comprehensive,
  up-to-date, and culturally tailored lactation services provided by
  trained physicians, nurses, lactation consultants, and
  nutritionists/dietitians.
- Establish hospital and maternity center practices that promote
  breastfeeding, such as the Ten Steps to Successful Breastfeeding.
- Develop breastfeeding education for women, their partners, and
  other significant family members during the prenatal and
  postnatal visits.

Workplace

- Facilitate breastfeeding or breast milk expression in the
  workplace by providing private rooms, commercial grade breast
  pumps, milk storage arrangements, adequate breaks during the
  day, flexible work schedules, and onsite childcare facilities.
- Establish family and community programs that enable
  breastfeeding continuation when women return to work in all
  possible settings.
- Encourage childcare facilities to provide quality breastfeeding
  support.

Family and Community

- Develop social support and information resources for breastfeeding women such as hotlines, peer counseling, and mother-to-mother support groups.
- Launch and evaluate a public health marketing campaign portraying breastfeeding as normal, desirable, and achievable.
- Encourage the media to portray breastfeeding as normal, desirable, and achievable for women of all cultures and socioeconomic levels.
- Encourage fathers and other family members to be actively involved throughout the breastfeeding experience.

Research

- Conduct research that identifies the social, cultural, economic, and psychological factors that influence infant feeding behaviors, especially among African American and other minority and ethnic groups.
- Improve the understanding of the health benefits of breastfeeding, especially in reducing the risk for chronic childhood diseases among disadvantaged infants and children.
- Monitor trends on the incidence and duration of exclusive, partial, and minimal breastfeeding, including minority and ethnic groups.
- Compare the cost-effectiveness of different programs that promote, protect, and support breastfeeding to ensure optimal use of resources.
- Conduct research to better understand the role of fathers in promoting breastfeeding.
- Evaluate the influence of brief postpartum hospital stays on the initiation and duration of breastfeeding.
- Determine the safety of over-the-counter and prescription products taken by lactating women on infant health.
- Conduct a large, well-designed case-control study on the effects of breast implants on childhood disorders.

INDEX